Professional Skills in Radiology

Practising as a radiologist is about more than image interpretation. *Professional Skills in Radiology* provides a concise handbook of essential non-interpretative skills a medical imaging doctor should possess. The book explores important professional development skills needed to work with diagnostic and procedural radiology patients, within healthcare multidisciplinary teams and in the community. It also provides a resource to bring together important concepts in evidence-based practice, research and quality assurance, medical education, advocacy and ethical practice, and cultural safety. *Professional Skills in Radiology* will be an excellent companion resource for training and consultant radiologists, containing practice questions to help prepare for fellowship/board examinations or interview panels.

Professional Skills in Radiology

Sally Ayesa

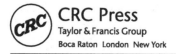

CRC Press
Taylor & Francis Group
Boca Raton London New York

CRC Press is an imprint of the
Taylor & Francis Group, an **informa** business

First edition published 2025
by CRC Press
2385 NW Executive Center Drive, Suite 320, Boca Raton FL 33431

and by CRC Press
4 Park Square, Milton Park, Abingdon, Oxon, OX14 4RN

CRC Press is an imprint of Taylor & Francis Group, LLC

ISBN: 978-1-032-73503-0 (hbk)
ISBN: 978-1-032-72684-7 (pbk)
ISBN: 978-1-003-46652-9 (ebk)

DOI: 10.1201/9781003466529

Typeset in Times
by SPi Technologies India Pvt Ltd (Straive)

For the doctors and future doctors who will be my medical imaging colleagues And for Imogen and Liam, who teach me more about life than can be found in any textbook.

Contents

Preface

Professionalism skills should be grown and practised, similar to any other clinical skill you develop in radiology. Just as we are not born able to read chest X-rays, we are not born excellent communicators, teachers, or team members. Instead, we hone these skills through repetition, making mistakes, and learning from them. It is not always comfortable, and being able to sit in this discomfort is part of the process.

Many of you reading this will be doing so in preparation for your radiology specialist exams. If so, I wish you luck in your studies, assessments, and the successful career that will undoubtedly follow. You inspired me to write this book.

When the Royal Australian and New Zealand College of Radiologists (RANZCR) released their new training program and exam structure in 2022, it included a new curriculum section titled 'Intrinsic Roles'. Too often downplayed as 'soft skills', these learning objectives covered those non-interpretive professional skills expected of qualified radiologists as they embarked on practice beyond training. Graduates must be effective communicators, inclusive collaborators, celebrated academics, ethical and productive researchers, and engaging teachers. We asked them to respect diversity in all its forms, exercise cultural competence throughout their practice, and embody the inclusive practice that came with it.

The creation of these competencies was modelled on the CanMEDs Framework created by the Royal College of Physicians and Surgeons of Canada. The model comprises of seven roles, which the clinician must develop to create the holistic clinician.

At its heart is the medical expert role, encompassing the knowledge and expertise a clinician gains over years of training, study and practice. Radiodiagnosis skills, clinical management, pathology, anatomy and physics are part of the medical expert domain. Surrounding this, there are six additional roles, which have formed the first six domains in the Intrinsic Roles syllabus:

- Communicator
- Collaborator
- Leader
- Health advocate
- Professional
- Scholar

The seventh group of outcomes relates to cultural competency, encompassing skills essential for delivering high-quality, inclusive patient care and working effectively within a medical imaging team.

In my former role as a Director of Radiology Training, however, I quickly found that while these learning objectives were important, they could have been better understood. Moreover, there was a sense that these graduate qualities should be inherently possessed or just common sense. The difficulty was that while these concepts were perceived as somewhat amorphous, our College would now examine them in an oral short-answer exam format.

As a writer of short answer examinations for several years, I know you must have a robust answer key for a standardised and fair assessment to support the question. This means that the examiner needs to have a clear understanding of the correct answer. By extension, if radiologists were going to prepare for questions on professionalism skills, they needed to get specific and start to think critically.

While sections of this book will have an Australian and New Zealand flavour, I have worked to include definitions and concepts broadly applicable to radiology practice worldwide. Professionalism is important no matter where you practise, and I know we share the same goal of delivering the best care possible to our patients. As you work through the book, you may like to take some moments to reflect on the differences and similarities between our health systems.

Research into professionalism skills spans industries, and you will notice that I have drawn concepts from the business world into our healthcare discussions. Each chapter references key literature, which I encourage you to explore should you wish to delve deeper. Hopefully, I have summarised the important concepts so you don't have to start from scratch.

The content covered is loosely guided by the learning objectives provided by the Australian and New Zealand College of Radiologists. I have taken the liberty of going beyond the RANZCR curriculum to explore departmental culture, leadership styles, and diversity, equity, and inclusion in greater depth. This is partly due to my interest in these topics, but it is also because I feel strongly that members of the medical imaging community should be involved in conversations around these themes. As a global radiology community, we owe it to ourselves to be informed so we can grow together.

I hope that this book serves as a useful guide to achieving success for those of you preparing for exams. Each section contains a few practice questions to help review the content and practise. In fact, writing these practice questions for my blog (becominga-radiologist.online) was the start of this book. If you are interested, check out the short section at the end of the book with my tips for preparing for radiology fellowship exams.

As a cis-gendered, white Australian woman, I do acknowledge my privilege. I have written about diversity, equity and inclusion, cultural competency and safety from my viewpoint, drawing from resources and literature to inform the discussion best. I accept my limitations and know that my unconscious bias is at play, but I know equally how important awareness and education around these topics are. As you read, I encourage you to reflect on your unconscious bias and how this impacts how you perceive the world as a clinician and individual.

For those of you picking up this book at the start of your radiology journey – welcome! I have included some more fundamental sections to help you, such as sections on patient flow in imaging departments and approaching the radiology report. Increasingly, interviews for radiology training positions will probe your knowledge of professional skills and current events in radiology. For those of you preparing to interview for a radiology training position, I hope this book will provide some context and fundamentals for the questions. At the end, there is a short section with tips for approaching radiology training applications and interviews.

A note on the terminology in this book. In my Australian practice I am qualified as both a clinical radiologist and a nuclear medicine specialist. While there is some overlap between the two specialties, they are distinct. Although I use the term 'radiologist' or 'medical imaging specialist' interchangeably throughout the book, any discussion of professional skills can be applied to radiology and nuclear medicine practice settings (with occasional tweaks). Also, consider any place where I say 'radiologist' to encompass both the specialist and the junior medical imaging doctor.

In Australia, junior doctors undertaking official radiologist training are called trainees or registrars. I have primarily used these terms to describe training radiologists throughout the book, but note that the names can vary. For example, in the USA, training radiologists are called radiology residents, and in the UK, they are called specialist registrars.

This guide is not comprehensive. It can't be. Like our understanding of medicine, our knowledge of how to deliver the highest-quality patient care, how to work best with each other, and how to learn, teach, and explore our subject constantly changes. Furthermore, as technology and our use of it evolves, so do we. It was not too long ago that radiology was read purely on film, and now we are amid the revolutionary rise of artificial intelligence. Use this knowledge as a basecoat and update it as you see fit. Practice is variable, and your own local policies and procedures will be unique.

While studying, I remember my textbooks being covered in brightly coloured annotations depicting the pearls I had picked up along the way. If that is how you learn best, I give you full permission to deface my words – in print or electronically.

A final word of advice, borrowed from *The Witcher III* – "Don't train alone, it only embeds your errors." Take the time to learn from, and with, each other. It is far too easy to retreat into solitude as a radiologist, but medicine is a team sport. Together, we make each other better.

Happy learning!
Sally (she/her)

This book has been written on the lands of the Dharug, Cammaraygal, Darkinjung, Yagambeh and Gadigal people. I pay my respects to the Elders of those lands, past, present and emerging.

Acknowledgement

This book was mostly written during 2024, one the most professionally and personally challenging years of my life so far. Writing and researching the topics contained within these pages has gifted me a chance to reflect and provided insights I may not have had otherwise. I had more than a few little 'eureka' moments along the way.

I want to thank the medical imaging departments and the people in them who trained and mentored me, including Royal North Shore Hospital Nuclear Medicine and Radiology Departments, Royal Prince Alfred Radiology, Prince of Wales and Sydney Children's Hospital Nuclear Medicine, and the Central Coast Department of Radiology and Nuclear Medicine. I want to thank not only the doctors but also the radiographers, nuclear medicine technologists, scientists, nurses and support staff who took the time to make me a better clinician and person.

Thank you to my colleagues at RANZCR, especially Dr Jane McEniery, for supporting the creation of this book from the outset. To the wonderful community of women mentors and heroes who are willing to have the hard conversations, especially Prof Catherine Jones, Dr Cathy Hayter and Dr Emmeline Lee. Thank you to Prof Stefan Tigges and Dr David Little for reviewing my proposal and supporting my endeavour from the other side of the world.

I also express my thanks to the registrars who took the time to read some of the chapters and provide feedback, including Dr Gemma Sheehan-Dare, Dr Claire Ephraums, Dr Alexander Dunn, Dr George Sidhom, Dr Christine Yang and Dr Ashvin Ragavan. I am grateful that you thought reading the drafts was a worthwhile use of your study or personal time. I know you will all make wonderful radiologists, and it is an honour to be part of your training journeys.

In 2023 I decided to do something different and complete a writing course. Thank you to the Faber Academy, Patti Miller and all the 'Checked Pants Writing Group' members for the support, feedback and insight. I know this isn't a memoir, but there are pieces of me in here. Particular thanks to Henry Chapman, who offered his edits and assistance in the final days of my pulling together the manuscript. Grammarly is indeed an excellent tool!

To my long-suffering PhD supervisors, Professors Stuart Grieve, Annette Katelaris, and Patrick Brennan: At the outset, you warned me not to be distracted by other things that would pop up along the way. I assured you that I would be fine, but since I have taken a left turn and written a book, it seems you were right all along. I'll get back to the project now.

Thank you to the University of Sydney Medical School for giving me an academic home. It is a privilege to be part of such an innovative faculty and to be given a chance to be part of the ongoing conversation about how we teach and learn medical imaging, and medicine more broadly. I still believe that working out how to teach radiology to first-year medical students is one of the hardest jobs I have, but I am immensely grateful that you allow me to do it.

To my virtual community of like-minded educators at Radiopaedia: I am still blown away that you brought me to the editorial board and are willing to let me talk to the world about everything from chest X-rays to gender diversity. I have learnt more about what it takes to reach an audience from you than anyone. Special thanks to Dr Andrew Dixon, Andrew Murphy, Prof Vikas Shah and Prof Frank Gaillard for your kindness and willingness to help me improve. Your feedback is always bang on.

Thank you to the team at CRC Press/Taylor & Francis Group for giving me the chance to write this book. Special thanks to my editor Shivangi Pramanik for her patience and support during the writing process.

To my friends and family, whose unwavering support over my entire medical career got me where I am today. They know me better than I know myself and are willing to put up with my idiosyncrasies and wild ideas. To Arwen, who always cheers me up with a meme when work, life, or both are getting on top of me.

Thank you to my parents, Sue and Don, and my sister Lucy for everything. A short paragraph is not enough to express my gratitude for what you have given to me, your son-in-law and my children.

To my husband Charlie, I would not have accomplished half the things I have without you by my side. Without you, things would be chaos, and I would forget breakfast most days. Thank you for your patience, understanding, and love. I know that I spent almost all of our holiday in Bali scrambling to get my manuscript finished, and I appreciate that you never once made me feel bad about it.

To my children, Imogen and Liam, you constantly inspire me, make me laugh, and bring me more joy and fulfilment than I thought possible. You both approach life with such courage, and I am honoured to be your mother.

Finally, to the next generation of radiologists and nuclear medicine specialists. I have been privileged to be a small part of some of your educational journeys already, and I hope I have the chance to continue that in the future. Thank you for inspiring this project. I look forward to working alongside you.

About the Author

Dr Sally Ayesa

Dr Sally Ayesa is a radiologist and nuclear medicine specialist from Sydney Australia, who loves to start conversations about radiology practice.

After completing her radiology training at Royal Prince Alfred and Royal North Shore Hospitals in Sydney, she went on to complete her nuclear medicine fellowship at Royal North Shore, Prince of Wales and Sydney Children's Hospitals. She received the prestigious HR Sear Medal for the best performance in the RANZCR Part II radiodiagnosis examination for 2017. Her clinical interests include chest radiology and oncology imaging, with a focus on lung cancer and prostate cancer imaging. She is a staff specialist at Royal North Shore Hospital.

Sally is the specialty lead for medical imaging at the University of Sydney Medical School, where she also works in academic support. She is completing a PhD in medical imaging education, considering how we can better educate medical students and non-radiologist clinicians about the fascinating specialties of radiology and nuclear medicine.

Sally is a member of the Radiopaedia editorial board, having co-convened the Radiopaedia Virtual Conference in 2022 and 2024. She is a member of the RANZCR Curriculum Assessment Committee, and a former member of the RANZCR Diversity, Equity and Inclusion Taskforce. Sally is currently part of the radiology team working towards implementing the National Lung Cancer Screening Program in Australia.

Communication and Conduct

1

FUNDAMENTALS OF COMMUNICATION

Effective communication is the foundation of high-quality clinical practice across health-care settings and specialties, and indispensable to any medical imaging professional. Well-developed communication is linked to improved patient outcomes, better patient satisfaction and reduced rates of medical errors.[1] Communication skills, as is the case with any other clinical or professional radiology skill, require practice and refinement.

Traditionally, radiology has been plagued by the stereotype of the isolated clinician, alone in a dark room, adverse to social interaction. In modern practice, the diversity of medical imaging means that radiologists or nuclear medicine clinicians can spend variable amounts of time in patient-facing capacities. An interventional radiologist may spend much of their day interacting directly with patients. In contrast, a radiologist reporting in a teleradiology or a remote capacity may interact with patients either sparingly or even not at all. Good communication will be essential regardless of your eventual practice setting or subspecialisation.

Communication types in radiology

Communication in radiology clinical settings can be divided into:[2]

- Verbal communication
- Non-verbal communication
- Visual communication

Verbal communication is not limited to oral interactions; it also encompasses the written word. For radiologists, this includes written radiology reports, diagnostic and procedural referrals, notes within the electronic medical record and exchanges between colleagues over cloud-based collaboration software such as Microsoft Teams®.

Non-verbal communication encompasses all that is not explicitly said. This includes physical behaviours such as eye contact, posture, gestures and auditory features such as tone of voice. These cues can help a clinician convey interest and build

DOI: 10.1201/9781003466529-1

a connection or, conversely, betray annoyance and frustration – risking the erosion of patient trust.

As radiologists, **visual communication** through medical imaging is an inherent aspect of our work. As such, the skill is highly developed and refined over years of practice. Other forms of visual communication encountered in radiology include physical aids such as signage, pamphlets and infographics, multimedia elements and educational materials such as slides and videos. They can be a mixture of text and images, usually designed to augment understanding and improve engagement. Understanding and effectively using these visual aids can enhance patient education and engagement and strengthen the principles of patient-centred care.

Building rapport and trust

Broadly, **rapport** is establishing a connection based on mutual understanding and respect. Rapport is not inherent and should not be expected to evolve organically in all patient–clinician relationships. Despite its acknowledgement as a pillar of person-centred communication and care, the specifics of how we build rapport remain indistinct. Our collective understanding of how we establish rapport could be divided into six categories:[3]

- **Interpersonal coordination** e.g. mutual agreement, engagement, interpersonal dynamics
- **Positivity** e.g. maintenance of attention and interest, understanding, demonstration of concern
- **Connector qualities** e.g. honesty, sympathy, empathy, trust
- **Talk/verbal** e.g. use and remembrance of personal details such as names, kind words, small talk
- **Non-verbal** e.g. eye contact, positional symmetry and physical mirroring, other non-verbal communication cues
- **Health profession-specific** e.g. conveyed professionalism, credibility, authenticity, respect for family members, willingness to admit limitations

Rapport is considered a prerequisite to gaining a patient's trust. **Trust** is "a set of expectations that the healthcare provider will do the best for the patient, and with goodwill, recognising the patient's vulnerability".[4] This trust can exist on a personal level, between individual healthcare professionals and patients, or on a larger scale where patients consider their faith in larger institutions (such as hospitals) and governing health bodies to deliver their care.

Establishing trust in a personal healthcare relationship is critical but inherently delicate due to the asymmetry of the relationship between patient and clinician responsible for their care.

Recent world events, including the COVID-19 pandemic and the associated actions of world and local governments, have been lived through a digital lens. The influences of social media and the dissemination of misinformation have contributed to an erosion of trust in healthcare for some patients. As such, people engage with and trust healthcare providers differently than in the past. Further information and assurances may be required during the rapport and trust-building phases of patient relationships to allow the successful delivery of care.

Person-centred care and communication

As mentioned earlier, depending on the area of practice within medical imaging, the time a radiologist spends in directly patient-facing environments is variable. An interventional radiologist may spend most of their day interacting with and managing patients, whereas a radiologist reporting remotely will have almost no direct patient interaction throughout their shift. However, just because the patient is not visible does not mean they should not remain at the forefront of the radiologist's mind as they interpret images and suggest management actions.

In **person-centred or patient-centred care models**, patients' attitudes, values, and preferences are central to the development of care plans and the provision of management.[5] This healthcare model correlates with improved patient outcomes, higher patient satisfaction levels, and more cost-effective service provision. The success of person-centred care relies on establishing mutually respectful relationships between healthcare providers and patients.

The person-centred approach requires careful communication with patients and relatives/carers (where appropriate) to understand unique care needs better and engage in shared decision-making. For patients in the imaging department specifically, the physical experience of undergoing an examination or imaging-guided procedure needs to be considered and balanced against the knowledge that the time within the department is a fraction of their overall care journey.

The facilitation of effective person-centred care hinges on the ability of the healthcare provider to engage in meaningful communication to build rapport. This rapport needs to be balanced against the requirement of radiology staff to glean the proper clinical information in a timely fashion so that service can continue or time-critical decisions can be made. Depending on the setting, radiological consultations may be brief and/or focused as necessary for the procedure or investigation about to be undertaken. Despite the relative brevity, patients need to feel heard and perceive actively participating in their care.[2, 6]

However, one of the challenges of communication in medical imaging is that patients usually seek general radiology services as part of a referral process at the behest of an external treating clinician. Patients visit for investigations or procedures requested by their primary treating doctor, to whom they will return for follow-up of results and further management. As such, radiologists must consider their role in the patient's overall care. While provisional results can be discussed in some circumstances (for example, a breast radiologist discussing the detection of a suspicious lesion that will require biopsy), delivery of formal results and sensitive conversations should, in most cases, be reserved for the patient's treating clinician. While there are some scenarios where the radiologist will be required to deliver bad news to a patient, this should be followed up by a formal review by their referring doctor (see *Chapter 1: Challenges In Patient Communication: Breaking bad news*).

Active listening

Active listening is a communication style that is honed over time. It goes beyond hearing the words that someone is saying, but attuning to non-verbal cues and responding with interest and empathy.[7] As the clinician in the conversation, the radiologist has two roles: eliciting the necessary clinical information and engaging and building rapport with the patient.

Active listening has three components:[8]

- Cognitive
- Emotional
- Behavioural

The **cognitive** aspect of active listening involves the clinician paying attention to the conversation. This includes recognising explicit information (answers to questions) and implicit information (non-verbal information). The radiologist must then synthesise explicit and implicit information to form their clinical assessment.

The **emotional** and **behavioural** aspects of active listening relate to the clinician's responses. Personal emotions must be balanced, aiming for a calm and compassionate demeanour throughout the interaction. Maintaining this demeanour can be difficult in certain circumstances, especially when the interaction involves an angry, aggressive, or distressed patient or requires the discussion of adverse or unexpected outcomes. The behavioural aspect requires the clinician to maintain a sense of interest and engagement within the interaction.

BOX 1.1   PRACTICE QUESTIONS

- Outline the importance of communication in providing high-quality person-centred care.
- Non-verbal communication is essential in establishing rapport with medical imaging patients. Briefly discuss this statement.

PATIENT ASSESSMENT, COUNSELLING AND CONSENT

Interventional radiology practice

Radiology was traditionally considered a service specialty that existed to support other medical specialties in providing care for their patients. While this remains true for diagnostic radiology and minor procedures, interventional radiology practice is evolving beyond a purely technical specialty. This means that modern interventional radiologists are more often engaged in the clinical consultive process and, at times, responsible for the patient's longitudinal care. The nature of this doctor–patient relationship varies as per local practice conventions and the skillset of the radiologist. This model of caring for more complex interventional radiology and neuroradiology patients is growing globally and will become increasingly commonplace. Similarly, some nuclear medicine specialists may be the primary managing clinician for patients undergoing treatment with radioisotopes for thyroid disease or malignancy.

Subspecialised interventional radiologists require the same imaging knowledge base as general radiologists but also need a greater depth of clinical expertise. This includes the management of medical therapies, pain, and other symptoms related to the condition they are treating. The interventional radiologist must have highly developed patient-facing communication skills and competency across outpatient clinics, inpatient management and multidisciplinary teams. The specialty is moving towards a model where the interventionalist directs all aspects of the patient's care until the patient's condition has resolved or evolved to the point that their input is no longer required.[1]

Patient flow in the imaging department

Patient and clinical flow through an imaging department will vary between practices, studies, and procedures. Figure 1.1 shows a simplified overview. Both diagnostic and procedural radiology start with a clinical referral and end with closing the communication loop back to the referring doctor. The final communication is most commonly through a written radiology report or letter.

Diagnostic imaging

Imaging referrals can be received in paper or electronic form. Some tests are booked directly, and some need radiographer or doctor review. Reviews often consider:

- Whether the clinical indication for the requested test is appropriate
- The urgency of the referral
- Whether any specific protocols are required to best answer the clinical question

Once a patient is assigned a booking time, they will be provided information regarding the logistics of the test and any specific preparation required, e.g., fasting or oral pre-hydration.

Some investigations require the completion of pre-screening checklists and consent forms, including magnetic safety forms for patients undergoing MRI scans or contrast screening and consent forms for patients planned for a CT scan with iodinated contrast. If the patient has technical or medical questions regarding the scan, administrative staff will connect them with the radiographers or doctors as appropriate.

Patients will be checked in on the day of arrival, and compliance with pre-preparation confirmed. If required, a cannula will be sited for intravenous contrast, and/or oral contrast will be provided.

Radiographers will escort the patient into the scanning room, where the images are acquired according to a standard or specified protocol. If additional imaging is required later in the day, the patient will be instructed to return.

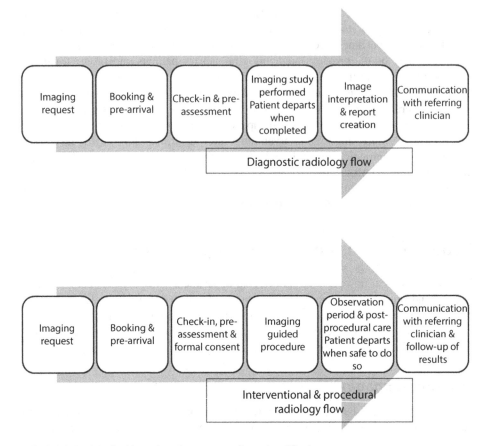

FIGURE 1.1   Medical imaging department flow simplified.

Once the study is completed, the radiographer, sonographer, or technologist reviews the images. If critically significant or uncertain findings are detected, a medical imaging clinician will be contacted for review. A repeat examination may be required if the study lacks technical adequacy or if a finding requires additional images.

If the scan is of good technical quality and the patient is safe, they leave the department and return to the care of their referring clinician. The radiologist will report the study and provide a report to the referrer.

At any point, the patient can request to speak with a doctor or revoke consent for the test.

Interventional/procedural radiology[1]

Patients may be referred for the procedure by a non-imaging clinician, or, increasingly, the interventionalists themselves may arrange the referral. A multidisciplinary team discussion may have already taken place for more complex patients.

Once an interventional procedure is requested, it will be reviewed by the clinical team. Appropriateness and final approval are granted based on:

- The clinical indication
- The patient's medical and surgical history
- The results of previous imaging (or procedural) studies
- Relevant results of other tests e.g. blood tests, histology

Depending on the nature and risks associated with the specific procedure, pre-test results and preparation may be required, such as:

- Blood tests e.g. coagulation studies, full blood counts, liver function or kidney function tests
- Antibiotic prophylaxis
- Diet or fasting regimes

Pre-consultation may occur in an outpatient clinic or on the day within the radiology department. The procedure will be explained, including the risks, benefits and limitations. The role of alternative diagnosis or management options may also be discussed to allow the patient to make an informed decision about the direction of their care. If the patient chooses to proceed, informed consent will be formally documented (see *Chapter 1: Patient Assessment, Counselling and Consent: Informed consent*). At this appointment, the radiologist may also:

- Revisit the clinical history
- Perform a targeted physical examination
- Review medications
- Document allergies
- Create, confirm or revise management plans

If anaesthesia or more complex sedation is required, the patient may also require clinical review by the anaesthetics team.

Nursing or other clinical staff will review the patient before the procedure, site cannulas if appropriate, and give any premedications.

Safety checklists and standard 'Time Out' protocols will occur before the procedure commences.

After the procedure, the patients will be monitored as per the guidelines for their specific procedure. If the patient is well enough to return home or be formally discharged, they will receive aftercare instructions. If the patient remains in the hospital, these instructions will be provided to the staff involved in their ongoing inpatient care.

Follow-up appointments may occur with the interventional radiology team or the referring clinician. At these appointments, any wound sites will be reviewed, stitches removed (if inserted), and results discussed. Referral for subsequent multidisciplinary team discussion may be required.

Consulting and assessing medical imaging patients

The clinical relationship and role of the medical imaging doctor within the patient's care will dictate the depth and nature of the initial consultation and whether subsequent review is required. The following section will focus primarily on typical interactions with patients in the medical imaging department, that is, those presenting for diagnostic imaging or procedures under the responsibility of an external clinician. These patient interactions proceed in a different – often abbreviated – fashion. While the interaction is limited by time in the context of a busy medical imaging practice, it is also limited by necessity and practicality. A 'long case' style medical history and examination will usually be excessive for the needs of the reporting radiologist.

While the review may be brief, it should not feel brusque, abrupt or confronting. Patients undergoing medical imaging tests frequently do so when they are unwell, frightened, vulnerable and/or uncertain. The imaging department is potentially an unfamiliar and confronting environment which can exacerbate these emotions. Clinicians need to consider this when interacting with patients, taking the time to allow them to ask questions, voice concerns, and seek clarification.

As medical imaging professionals, we often take for granted how poorly understood the fields of radiology and nuclear medicine are to the public. Taking the time to address a patient's questions and misconceptions has high potential value.

Reviewing diagnostic imaging requests

The starting point, and often the primary source of information about the patient, is the imaging referral written by the requesting clinician. It is customary to consider that scans are *requested* for patients rather than *ordered* for a patient. This respects the authority of the specialist radiologist to review the patient documentation and determine whether the imaging study requested is the most appropriate course of action for the stated indication.

Medical imaging requests should give enough information about the clinical presentation and the patient's background medical history to allow the reviewing clinician (or radiographer or support staff) to clearly understand the purpose of the examination and provide enough information to formulate an accurate report. Requests should include major diagnoses that could impact the imaging interpretation, such as a history of cancer, major surgery or other chronic illness.

BOX 1.2   FOR EXAMPLE ...

A 60-year-old patient is referred for a CT of the chest. The request form states:

"Cough ?lower respiratory tract infection".

The scan reveals multiple pulmonary nodules, which are suspicious for metastatic cancer.

If this was an unexpected finding, it represents the diagnosis of a severe illness with potentially devastating consequences. The reporting radiologist would pause

---

the flow of reporting to call the treating team to discuss the findings and/or review the medical record to gather more information about the patient.

If the patient were *known* to have pulmonary metastatic disease before the investigation, additional phone calls and review of the records would not have needed to take place – saving the reporting radiologist time and avoiding the interruption.

In the same vein, imaging requests should indicate the presence and location of prior imaging, especially if it has been performed at a secondary site. Diagnostic accuracy and value are higher when comparison imaging is available to contextualise imaging findings or better inform diagnostic certainty.

If further information is required, the radiologist, trainee or representative should contact the referring clinician for clarification. The electronic medical record and prior scans should be reviewed as required (if available), guided by the case's complexity.

Targeted patient consultation and assessment

While direct clinician review of patients is uncommon in diagnostic imaging (except for instances of clinical concern or unexpected findings), it is expected before interventional radiology procedures and some nuclear medicine studies. It is important to remember that medical imaging is usually a referral-based service and that the treating team/referring clinician is the primary responsibility for the patient and their follow-up.

Management of acutely unwell or deteriorating patients varies between hospital-based and community practices. In hospitals, acutely unwell inpatients should be discussed with their treating team, with calls to the medical emergency team (e.g. Code Blue) called in cases where immediate help is required. Outpatients attending a medical imaging department needing urgent review should be directed to the care of their referring doctor or the emergency department. Similarly, in community practice, an urgent review of the patient by their referring or local doctor should be arranged, with an ambulance transfer to the hospital in cases requiring emergent care. In all cases, adequate verbal handover should be provided to the clinician who referred the patient for the imaging study.

The initial consultation aims to gain a general understanding of the patient's medical context and gather relevant additional information on the specific medical condition being investigated or managed. When taking a history in radiology or nuclear medicine, the conversation should be targeted towards the clinical history of the presentation and screening for other significant diagnoses or surgery that may impact how the test or procedure is performed/interpreted.

BOX 1.3   FOR EXAMPLE ...

A patient presents for a nuclear medicine bone scan to investigate low back pain.

Clinicians will protocol the scan based on the most likely cause e.g. facet joint arthritis, skeletal infection or malignancy. A study looking for infection or inflammation will require both early and delayed phase imaging, whereas a malignancy screening needs delayed phase imaging alone.

A targeted musculoskeletal history is taken to determine whether prior injuries, surgeries, or conditions may cause abnormal imaging findings on the scan. A brief screen for major illnesses and medical history is also helpful. Knowing this information will improve the diagnostic certainty when the images are interpreted.

Patients should also be asked if they have had prior imaging studies and where they were performed.

The test should be explained and written or verbal consent confirmed.

BOX 1.4   FOR EXAMPLE ...

A patient presents for a CT-guided lung biopsy.

The clinical review will start with a brief conversation about how the lesion was found and any associated symptoms the patient may have. A short discussion about how the patient feels is helpful in screening for new signs or symptoms.

A targeted thoracic history should be taken, including assessment for underlying lung diseases, smoking history or thoracic surgery. Eliciting whether the patient becomes breathless or experiences pain while lying down will be important in deciding the optimal positioning of the patient on the CT table.

Assessment of bleeding risk (including predisposing conditions or anticoagulant medications) is pertinent (as with any procedure) as it will influence whether and how the procedure is performed and impact the informed consent process.

The proceduralist would have ideally reviewed comparison/recent imaging before the patient's arrival. Images will be re-reviewed on the day and used in planning.

The procedure should be explained, and written informed consent should be confirmed.

Counselling patients before procedures

As part of the consultation, the procedure should be discussed with the patient and their support person or legal guardian, if applicable. This should start with an explanation of what to expect and how the procedure is performed. Information should be presented in clear, accessible language without jargon. The rationale for the procedure in the context of the patient's clinical presentation should be clearly explained and balanced against the risk of adverse events and complications. If appropriate, alternative diagnostic or therapeutic options should be discussed with the patient and compared with the planned interventional radiology procedure. This step reinforces person-centred care, preserving autonomy in the decision-making process. Finally, the patient should be invited to ask questions of the radiologist.[1]

Completing the counselling process should provide the patient with adequate information to engage with the informed consent process. For more complex elective procedures with higher-risk profiles, patients should ideally be given at least one day to consider the information provided before they are invited to provide informed consent.

Informed consent

Informed consent represents a person's decision to proceed with a treatment, procedure or intervention as part of their healthcare plan. The decision is made by the person voluntarily, following the provision of accurate and relevant information regarding the risks and benefits of the management plan, considering any alternative options. It is the onus of the healthcare provider to ensure that the person making the decision has adequate knowledge and understanding, inviting questions and clarification as needed.[9]

If adequate information has not been provided to the patient before proceeding or they cannot comprehend it, the consent may be invalid. A qualified interpreter is required if the patient does not have adequate English language proficiency to fully understand the information being provided. Medico-legally, family members should not act as interpreters for formal consent (see *Chapter 1: Challenges in Patient Communication: Communicating with patients with limited fluency in English*). It is the clinician's responsibility to ensure that all reasonable attempts have been made to assist the patient in understanding the information provided, including helping them overcome language, cultural or ability barriers to their understanding.

For the consent to be considered valid, four criteria must be met:[10]

- The patient giving consent must have the capacity to do so (see below)
- Consent must be given voluntarily and freely
- Consent must be specific to the investigation, procedure or treatment discussed
- Consent must be informed by adequate information

For patients undergoing diagnostic scans or imaging-guided procedures, the full informed consent process is usually shared between the referring clinician(s) and the radiologist.[11] This is because the referring clinician usually has a more comprehensive knowledge of the patient's care, and the radiologist has a more thorough knowledge of the investigation or procedure. As such, clear and transparent communication (verbal or written) should occur between clinicians to ensure that the consent process has been upheld. The radiologist should be available for consultation and advice if referrers need assistance understanding the investigation/procedure to counsel their patient and/or for educational purposes.

Even if the referring clinician has completed the written consent process (or the patient has completed it before arriving), the clinician or radiographer performing the investigation or procedure should confirm consent, inviting further questions and clarifications and reiterating information as needed.

Types of informed consent

There are three methods of providing informed consent:[11]

- Implied consent
- Verbal consent
- Written consent

All three types of consent require the person to have been provided adequate information to allow them to make an informed decision; however, how this consent is formalised depends on the practice setting, the risk profile of the intervention and the nature of the procedure.

Implied consent occurs when a patent indicates their agreement through actions, e.g., complying voluntarily with the radiographer's instructions as they are prepared for a chest X-ray.

Verbal consent is provided when a person vocalises their agreement to proceed following a discussion with the healthcare provider. This agreement should be documented in the patient's medical record.

Written consent is required for interventions and procedures that are more complex and/or invasive and have recognised adverse risks or potential side effects. Written consent is also required for studies and procedures performed as part of a research protocol. Many imaging departments have dedicated consent forms, requiring documentation of the investigation/procedure and relevant risks and benefits, with the clinician and patient countersigning the document.

Capability to provide informed consent

The key to providing informed consent relies on the person's ability to understand the information provided so that they can use it to make a decision regarding their health (or the health of another). Specifically, they need to:[9]

- Understand the facts surrounding the investigation/procedure
- Understand the alternative treatment options available
- Understand how the potential consequences could affect them (including whether they chose to proceed or not to proceed)
- Weigh up the options with their risks and benefits (including the risks/benefits of not consenting)
- Retain the information provided by the healthcare team and recall details
- Communicate their decision and personal understanding to healthcare providers

Reasons why a patient may be unable to provide informed consent include:

- Young age (with ages of consent and definitions of 'mature minors' dependent on local jurisdictions)
- Intellectual disability or other cause of reduced mental capacity
- Emergencies where the patient is sedated/anaesthetised or has a reduced level of consciousness

The inability to provide informed consent may be temporary, for example, in sedated/anaesthetised patients or patients with temporarily reduced mental capacity in the setting of acute illness.

Specific local legislation may impact one's capacity to consent. A patient being treated under a *Mental Health Act* is one such example.

Refusing and revoking consent

Patients who can provide informed consent for an investigation/procedure are medico-legally allowed to refuse consent. Similarly, people can revoke their consent at any time before or during an intervention (provided they are in a position to communicate). Should a patient verbally express their wish to revoke consent, the healthcare provider must cease even if a signed consent form has been completed. If appropriate, the reasons for withdrawing consent should be discussed, and the risks and benefits of ceasing or continuing should be revisited.

Suppose a patient with the capacity to consent chooses to withdraw that consent. After discussing this decision with the patient, the radiologist should communicate it with the referring clinician. It should be documented clearly in the written diagnostic or procedural report and/or patient medical record.

Managing complications and adverse events

An **adverse event** is defined by CIRSE (the Cardiovascular and Interventional Radiological Society of Europe) as "any unfavourable or unintended sign (including laboratory findings), symptom, or disease temporally associated with the use of a medical treatment or procedure that may or may not be considered related to the treatment or procedure".[1] A **complication** more specifically indicates when an unintended harm has resulted from the procedure, which may or may not impact the clinical course of the patient.[12] Adverse events are an inevitable but unwelcome part of medical imaging practice, despite the best efforts of individuals, departments and broader healthcare networks to minimise the risk of them occurring.

A three-step approach has been suggested for handling adverse events and complications in radiology:[12]

- Recognising
- Managing
- Learning

A complication or adverse event may be **recognised** during or after the procedure. Complications during the procedure are usually immediately apparent and can be managed on the spot with additional procedural steps. Post-procedural events can be more challenging to recognise and manage, although the majority will manifest within 24 hours after the procedure is completed. Post-procedure review (e.g., ward rounds, clinic visits, or phone calls) and the provision of clear patient information improve the chance of recognising these complications after the fact.

Ideally, a complication or adverse event should be addressed as quickly as possible. The specific steps taken and staff involved in the **management** are determined by the nature of the event, the perceived risk to the patient, and the radiologist's experience.

After the fact, a **learning** process should be undertaken to minimise or reduce the risk of the adverse event occurring again. Processes include mortality and morbidity meetings (M&M meetings) and peer-review/peer-feedback processes. Depending on the severity of the complication or adverse event, more in-depth investigation may be required (see *Chapter 3: Quality Improvement and Audit*).

A practice of 'open disclosure' or a 'legal duty of candour' is a standard inclusion within health policy worldwide. Such policies formalise the steps a medical staff member or team must take when communicating and managing patients inadvertently harmed during their medical care. Conversations following an adverse event/complication are often sensitive and the patient is vulnerable. Ideally, these discussions should be held in a quiet and private setting, with the patient offered the presence of a support person. If required, interpreter services should be arranged. Accurate medical records should be completed following the discussion.

The practice of open disclosure can (and should) involve:[13]

- **Acknowledgement** of the event to the patient (ideally within 24 hours), with the conversation recognising the seriousness of what has occurred
- An **apology** to the patient (and support persons), which explicitly uses the word "sorry"
- Provision of honest, transparent and timely ongoing **communication** to the patient (and support persons if required) and delivery of **care** on an ongoing basis as necessary
- Provision of appropriate **support** to staff involved in the incident

The process ideally involves a multidisciplinary team and adopts an integrated approach to improving patient safety. The radiology team should not undertake the open disclosure process in isolation, but involve different clinical and corporate groups as required. In many facilities, it also requires engagement with incident reporting systems and escalation/management as per local policies.

BOX 1.5   PRACTICE QUESTIONS

- The radiographers call you to review a scan while the patient is still on the CT table. The images demonstrate a life-threatening diagnosis. The patient is an outpatient. How would you approach this?
- Define informed consent and outline its importance in clinical radiology.
- Outline the principles for managing an adverse event, using the example of large volume post-procedural haemorrhage following CT-guided liver biopsy.

THE WRITTEN RADIOLOGY REPORT

Written reports represent the primary correspondence between the reporting radiologist and the clinician (or team of clinicians) responsible for a patient's care. As such, they must communicate crucial clinical information clearly and succinctly so clinical teams can act without confusion. It is also worthwhile noting that patients will often read their own radiology reports. As such, it is important to consider the implications of particular turns of phrase (e.g. cancer) and provide diagnostic and management recommendations with care.

At its most basic, the report summarises pertinent imaging findings as read by the reviewing radiologist, with an accompanying interpretation of these findings in the patient's clinical context. This definition, however, underplays the role of the radiologist's expertise and the potential value they add to patient care. Beyond simple detection of findings within the images, a radiologist's role is to synthesise findings, gain a greater understanding of the patient's condition and use this information to provide clinically useful diagnostic information and management recommendations. These insights are packaged into a clear and accessible communique to assist in further care.

As with other clinical and professional skills, report-writing aptitude builds over time, supported by one's evolving clinical knowledge and professional expertise. This continual development is necessary to match the changing nature of the discipline of imaging itself, with constant innovations in technology and service delivery and our constantly improving knowledge of disease processes and best clinical practice.

The initial development of reporting skills for training radiologists is variable. Structured education aimed at the approach reporting is not standardised, with many trainees learning through a mixture of apprentice-style observation, mentorship, review of corrections, and self-directed study. Module-style e-learning is accessible to some trainees to build fundamental knowledge, and some sites provide variable-length didactic sessions through orientation.

Reviewing the context of the study

Before describing findings, the front matter of the report should be reviewed so that the radiologists can familiarise themselves with the patient, check that the correct patient has undergone the correct procedure, and mentally map out a plan for reviewing the images.

Reviewing the referral

The clinical history and the scan modality/protocol will be intimately linked; that is, the examination or procedure should be able to provide insight into the clinical question posed. Further clinical information may need to be sought from the medical record or referrer.

The reporting style used will vary between imaging modalities and clinical indi-cations. For example, X-ray reports are usually brief and lack a separate conclusion, whereas cross-sectional reports for CT and MRI studies are more in-depth and technical.

Considering the patient's care context is also essential in framing the approach to the radiology report and has implications for interpreting images and providing manage-ment recommendations. Patients referred by a general practitioner from the community usually require more prescriptive management guidance than would be the case in a referral from an orthopaedic surgeon requesting imaging to assist with planning fracture management, for example.

Each report needs to include the clinical history for clinical and medico-legal purposes. The clinician provides this information in the referral letter, and the word-ing should be dictated as closely as possible. Any additional clinical information gleaned from patient interviews and/or sought from the medical record should also be recorded.

Comparison imaging and scan technique

A specific statement should be made regarding the existence and availability of compar-ison studies, listing the most relevant comparison investigations and/or the most recent if multiple serial studies are available for review. For each comparison investigation, the report should include the type of study (modality, contrast phase if relevant), the date it was performed and where it was performed (particularly important if the study was conducted at an external practice).

The reporting of the scan technique will vary according to the imaging modality used. As a rule, the technique statement should indicate the imaging modality and body region that has been imaged. Any contrast administration should be documented, includ-ing the route, e.g. intravenous iodine contrast or gadolinium, oral contrast, or rectal contrast.

For CT studies, the phase of contrast should be documented (e.g. non-contrast, arte-rial or portal venous phase). For MRI studies, the phases acquired should be listed. Techniques for ultrasound studies only need to be recorded if consent was required (e.g. transvaginal ultrasound) or the protocol is not standard. In nuclear medicine and PET, details of the radiopharmaceutical delivered, dosage, the type of images acquired, their timing, and the scan field of view should be included. Note, in nuclear medicine, the types of studies performed and individual protocols are highly variable.

Occasionally, the imaging protocol may be altered by the radiologist or radiogra-pher from that requested, for example due to unforeseen patient factors or unexpected findings. This should also be clearly documented with the justification for why the amendment occurred.

Protocol details are important medico-legally and convey important information to the referring clinician and future radiologists reporting studies for the patient. Each modality, sequence, and contrast phase has inherent advantages and disadvantages. As such, the accuracy of diagnosing and assessing a particular pathology varies based on the study technique.

Documenting adverse events and complications

If any adverse events or complications occurred during the investigation, this should be clearly documented within the technique or elsewhere in the report format. In addition to a brief summary of the event, any management steps, patient counselling and recommendations should be covered. Details often require reiteration within the report conclusion if there are current or future management implications e.g. contrast allergy, requirement for sedation for an MRI.

Imaging findings

While the art of systematic imaging interpretation is beyond the scope of this book, the approach to recording the detected findings is one of the most critical aspects of communication for the radiologist. The imaging findings typically comprise the majority of the report volume, with the length varying depending on the complexity of the study protocol and the pathology demonstrated. It is usually referred to as the body of the report.

Imaging findings should be presented clearly and logically, with the report structure tailored to the individual patient and examination. This section of the report should primarily focus on documentation of the scan findings, reserving imaging interpretation, opinion, and management for the report conclusion. Descriptions should be comprised of **true statements**, reflecting only what is seen and avoiding inference or extrapolation.

Observations should be listed briefly, with sparing use of perception terms such as "is demonstrated" or "is noted". If reporting with a narrative style (see *Reporting styles* section below) there may be a role for these sentence fragments to maintain stylistic flow and readability; however, overuse can lead to excessive words and, conversely, a lack of clarity.[14] The same principle applies to sentence structure. It is best to avoid long sentences with multiple conjunctions and clauses.

The dictation of imaging findings should follow an organised pattern so that the clinician reading the report can follow the written report to a logical conclusion without confusion.

The clinical question should be addressed clearly (ideally early) in the report and signposted so the clinician can easily find the relevant information. In the same vein, critical findings should be presented clearly and upfront, rather than 'buried' within the report.

Should a specific pathology be present, this should be reviewed in its entirety before moving on. For example, if a suspicious lung lesion is identified, the characteristics of the lesion should be described comprehensively e.g. size, enhancement characteristics, borders and relationship to surrounding structures. A report which identifies a pathology without adding characterisation offers little value to the clinician.

Guidance on the volume and nature of details to be included can be found in published classification systems, which exist for a wide range of diagnoses and pathologies. Consider the information that a clinician needs to direct management decisions if in doubt.

Beyond this, clinically relevant positive and negative findings should be reported clearly and systematically. Report clarity is improved by describing findings logically, which often mirrors the radiologist's systematic search pattern. For example, a description of hepatic findings will be followed by biliary tree findings, followed by a review of the pancreas and other upper abdominal organs.

When the initial dictation of the imaging observations has been completed, the text should be proofread for grammar and clarity. The report's structure should be adjusted as necessary, particularly if unexpected findings or additional associated pathologies need to be showcased.

Minimising diagnostic errors

In diagnostic radiology, errors can be divided into two groups: misses and misinterpretations. A **miss** is when a clinically significant finding is not detected and a **misinterpretation** is when there is an error in the interpretation of the finding, resulting in an incorrect diagnosis.[15] Different cognitive biases can potentially lead to diagnostic errors, even for experienced radiologists. These include:[15]

- **Anchoring bias:** failing to adjust a preliminary impression despite new evidence against it
- **Confirmation bias:** preferentially seeking information to confirm a pre-existing hypothesis
- **Satisfaction of report:** generating an impression based on the prior report rather than the current interpretation of imaging findings
- **Framing bias:** drawing different conclusions from the same data under the influence of how it is presented
- **Attribution bias:** assigning imaging findings or diagnoses to a patient based on stereotypes or other social, gendered or cultural biases
- **Satisfaction of search:** decreased diagnostic awareness or perceptiveness following the detection of a significant abnormality (see below)
- **Premature closure:** accepting a provision or working diagnosis as final before all information is considered
- **Inattention bias:** missing findings present in plain sight due to an unexpected or unfamiliar location or imaging appearance
- **Hindsight bias:** retrospective devaluation of the diagnostic difficulty of the imaging diagnosis

Satisfaction of search is a common source of error encountered when the reader consciously or unconsciously ceases their search after finding a primary abnormality. This premature disengagement can lead to missing an additional finding. Even though the reader goes through the motions of reviewing the images (sometimes even looking right at the abnormality), their perception is reduced, and the finding is not consciously detected.

A well-known study looking at perception when reading CT scans asked viewers to count lung nodules and then hid a picture of a gorilla in a single slice within one of the studies.[16] Only 4 of 24 radiologists reviewing the CT detected the gorilla, despite many looking right at it. This study demonstrated the phenomenon of **inattentional**

blindness. The radiologists (and other readers – none of whom found the gorilla) were focused on counting white lung nodules rather than looking for a black gorilla. Inattentional blindness also considers that individuals are less likely to detect an abnormality if they have not seen it before.

Employing comprehensive **search patterns** can minimise the risk of diagnostic errors. For plain X-rays, having a search pattern ensures that your eyes have looked over all parts of the image, increasing the chance of detecting an abnormality should it be there. Felson proposed one such approach for reading chest X-rays, which does just this:[17] urging the viewer to cast their eyes peripherally, move down the mediastinum, look at the lungs twice (they are the hero of the chest X-ray, after all), and then consider review areas.

For cross-sectional imaging, imaging review is more in-depth and requires moving between reconstructed planes (e.g. axial, sagittal, coronal) and changing the viewing windows to accentuate different tissue types.

When reviewing a stack of images in a series, the two primary review methods are scanning and drilling. In **scanning** techniques, each slice is examined before moving to the next one. In **drilling** techniques, the eye is trained on a specific area (e.g. the right anterior half of the lungs). The stack of images is scrolled through with the eyes fixed on this point. This is repeated for each anatomical area being reviewed. Drilling techniques are quicker than scanning and have been shown to reduce the number of diagnostic errors.[18] Diagnostic radiologists typically favour this approach.

Reporting styles

There are several different reporting styles which radiologists use individually or in combination:

- Narrative style
- Structured reporting
- Templates

Narrative style reporting is the traditional approach to report creation, where descriptions are free-flowing prose. This style is anecdotally the most common and is favoured by many radiologists as it is easily tailored to the individual patient and reporting flow. It also reflects the traditionally held value of the 'art' of the radiology report as a verbal manifestation of the radiologist's image reading and interpretation style. However, a purely narrative approach has drawn recent criticism for its style, structure and formatting variability. There are concerns narrative style is more likely to lack clarity, and has a greater risk of omitting important associated findings leading to misinterpretation.

Structured reporting has a broad definition and is sometimes called 'standardised' or 'template' reporting. It is commonly utilised for complex examinations, modalities and pathologies with clear reporting guidelines, and studies with a clear progression or checklist approach, e.g., upper abdominal ultrasound.

The prescriptiveness of structured reporting varies widely, from a subheading approach with narrative or free-text descriptions to a more rigid text-selection format.

For a CT study covering multiple body regions, the report can be broken into sub-headings to arrange narrative descriptions. For example:

- Brain
- Head and neck
- Thorax
- Abdomen & pelvis
- Musculoskeletal

In addition, some pathologies that affect multiple organ systems but are part of a single unifying diagnosis have a standard reporting structure to allow more streamlined communication between radiologists and the treating team. In oncology, for example, reporting of solid organ cancers usually follows a standard report with the following (or similar) headings:

- Primary tumour
- Lymph nodes
- Metastases
- Other findings

Template reporting is now commonplace for some specific studies or for the assessment of specific imaging findings; however, its use is ultimately guided by the preferences of the imaging practice and reporting radiologist. It is a more prescriptive form of structured reporting, where standard structure and phrases are auto-populated by the reporting software, and the radiologist adds relevant phrasings and additional findings as needed. For example, MRI prostate studies are routinely reported in their entirety to align with the ACR PI-RADS guidelines.[19] Thyroid nodules are often individually described and reported in line with ACR TI-RADS guidelines,[20] with the checklist-style assessment incorporated into the comprehensive thyroid ultrasound report.

The checklist approach to template reporting helps present information clearly and succinctly while still providing comprehensive information for diagnosis and guiding clinical management.[21] Structured reports can also be useful guides for trainees and radiologists less familiar with the imaging test. Other benefits include standardising reporting lexicon and assessment, reducing transcription errors, and ensuring greater adherence to guidelines and society recommendations for specific lesion assessment.

The greatest concern amongst radiologists regarding the template approach is rigidity, particularly when reporting more complex cases.[21] There is also a perception that rigid reporting structures diminish individual expression and can negatively impact the clarity and readability of the study. Conversely, the error rate may increase if there is over-reliance on the template to guide image review, particularly for inexperienced training radiologists. The impact of integrating templates into the reporting software is also a consideration, mainly if there is an inability to add free text or change descriptions to convey the findings as they relate to the individual case.

TABLE 1.1 Standardised lexicon to describe diagnostic certainty.

REPORT PHRASE	HOW CERTAIN THE RADIOLOGIST IS
Consistent with ...	>90%
Suspicious for ...	
Probably ...	~75%
Possibly ...	~50%
... less likely	~25%
Unlikely ...	<10%

Adapted from Oladele & Puzi.[22]

Conveying diagnostic certainty

How radiologists indicate the certainty of their provisional diagnoses in the medical imaging report varies widely. This has prompted groups to propose that certain phrases within the radiology report should correspond to specific degrees of diagnostic certainty. The model proposed by Panicek and Hricak correlates particular phrases with the approximate level of certainty of the reporting clinician[22] (Table 1.1).

BOX 1.6   FOR EXAMPLE ...

You are reporting a CT chest; you detect a lung mass. You notice it has the classic aggressive imaging features of primary lung cancer, with enlarged hilar and mediastinal lymph nodes and a few lytic skeletal lesions.

You are highly confident that this person has metastatic lung cancer and conclude the report as:

"Imaging findings as consistent with metastatic cancer secondary to a right lower lobe primary lung cancer."

BOX 1.7   FOR EXAMPLE ...

You are reporting a follow-up CT scan for a patient with treated melanoma. There is a borderline enlarged lymph node in the axilla which has increased in size from previously.

You are not sure whether it could be inflammatory or related to the cancer - it would be a 'coin flip' or 50/50 chance. In this report, you describe the node as:

"A borderline enlarged left axillary lymph node is possibly reactive or neoplastic..."

You conclude the report with your recommendations for how the referring clinician could address this further.

Terms can be used in combination to rank differential diagnoses and convey your preferences. For example, a patient has been referred for lower abdominal pain and a CT abdomen and pelvis is arranged. The patient has severe diverticulosis, which has given the sigmoid colon a thickened appearance. You believe that the diagnosis is most likely chronic sigmoid diverticulitis but know that the diagnosis of exclusion in these cases is a large bowel cancer. The conclusion could be phrased as "Circumferential thickening of the large bowel is *probably* related to chronic sigmoid diverticulitis, with a neoplastic lesion considered *less likely*."

In conclusion ...

The final paragraph of the medical imaging report is known by several different names, including 'Conclusion', 'Impression', or 'Comment'. Regardless of its title, it serves the same purpose – to summarise the study findings/diagnoses and document management recommendations clearly and concisely. If the referring clinician was contacted to discuss the case this is documented at the end of the report.

The report's conclusion is essentially a synthesis of all that has come before, repackaged to address the clinical question specifically and alert the medical team to any additional clinically significant findings. While we would like to believe that the referrer reviews the entirety of the report, they may only look at the conclusion in reality. As such, it is essential to get it right.

Fundamental principles for the creation of a clear and helpful impression include:[14]

- Leading with the diagnosis, supported by a summary of the relevant key findings, which will improve the understanding of the diagnosis and impact management
- Using accessible medical language that avoids technical radiology jargon and is clearly understood by the non-radiologist clinician
- Avoidance of redundancy and restating description from the body of the report
- Avoidance of clinically insignificant findings which do not require management or monitoring
- Providing appropriate management recommendations (when appropriate)

Management recommendations will vary according to the practice context and the referring clinician. For example, a general practitioner may need more guidance regarding additional imaging tests and clinical follow-up than a specialist surgeon.

A commonly used (and often-overused) phrase in radiology reports is "Clinical Correlation Recommended". This phrase can sometimes be perceived as condescending (of course, clinicians will consider the patient context when interpreting the radiology report) and unhelpful as it does not provide specific information about what to review or how to proceed. If specific correlation is genuinely required, it is best to be clear as to the nature of this, for example:

- Correlation with liver function tests is recommended
- Correlation with clinical signs of gastro-oesophageal reflux is recommended
- Correlation with point tenderness is recommended

- Correlation with abdominal examination findings is recommended
- Correlation with a history of trauma is recommended

Communicating life-threatening or clinically significant findings

Clinically significant or life-threatening findings may be detected during or immediately after the study is acquired (e.g., by the supervising radiologist or scanning radiographer) or at the time of final reporting.

How quickly these findings need to be communicated to the managing team is determined by their severity. For example, the detection of an acute aortic dissection needs to be immediately discussed with the referring clinician, as any delay in treatment may prove fatal for the patient. Incidental detection of a malignancy will still require discussion with the referring team, although this can be delayed until the radiologist is done crafting the report.

If communication between the reporting radiologist and the referring team occurs, this should be clearly documented at the conclusion of the report. This includes who findings were conveyed to and the time and date the exchange took place, e.g., *Findings discussed with Dr Brown at 12pm, 1ˢᵗ January 2025.*

Direct two-way communication is preferable but not always practical. If electronic or other one-way communication has occurred, it may be pertinent to document this as well, e.g., *Voice message left for Dr Brown at 12 p.m. on January 1, 2025.*

BOX 1.8   PRACTICE QUESTIONS

- Discuss the use of structured reporting in radiology, comparing the benefits and potential limitations.
- Outline the importance of conveying the level of diagnostic certainty you have in your reports, considering the potential impact on clinical outcomes.
- The radiographers call you to review a scan that appears to demonstrate a new diagnosis of incidental metastatic disease. How would you manage this?
- Describe the key elements of safe handover of care between medical imaging and clinical teams when a clinically significant abnormality has been detected in a diagnostic study.

RESOURCES AND PATIENT INFORMATION

A range of resources exist to help educate patients about medical imaging investigations and procedures at different stages of their journey. The target audience often extends beyond patients and their carers to referring clinicians and other non-radiological medical colleagues. For example, resources may be designed to:

- Help patients decide whether an interventional procedure is right for them before confirming their booking
- Outline what to expect from a practical perspective
- Itemise the preparation required before arriving for an appointment

Government organisations, national imaging societies, the local health system, or imaging departments may develop resources to meet specific patient needs. Examples include pamphlets and fact sheets (printed or electronic), wall posters, websites, or multimedia productions such as short videos.

Pre- and post-procedure resources

Preparation resources are important for patients undergoing imaging-guided procedures and more complex imaging tests to help them understand the rationale for the procedure, what to expect, and the risks vs benefits. Most commonly, this information is available in pamphlet style, either as a physical copy or, more commonly, in digital form, which can be emailed to the patient directly or accessed through the internet.

Information presented in other digital media forms, such as websites or short videos, can supplement pamphlets. Practice-specific resources developed by specialist societies or healthcare organisations are ideally complementary.

Well-designed and well-received patient preparation resources are presented in clear print and plain language, which is easily understood by non-medical members of the public.[23] Resources need to be linguistically accessible to people across a broad range of education and health literacy levels, as well as variable cultural and ethnic backgrounds. Ideally, resources should be available in a variety of languages or medical imaging staff should be able to direct patients to where to find those resources. Resources should also be accessible to patients with physical disabilities such as hearing or visual impairment.

Online radiology resources for patients

Online collections of patient and clinician resources are now commonplace on the internet, often developed by large imaging societies or subspecialty interest groups. These resources are usually designed to:

- Provide current and accurate information on medical imaging services to health consumers and potential referring clinicians
- Improve communication between radiology services, referring clinicians, their patients and support people
- Showcase the role that radiology can play in the management of certain conditions
- Increase awareness of and engagement with medical imaging

Including clinician-specific and patient/consumer-specific resources in collections is useful, as it allows the adjustment of technical language and provides more targeted information regarding both groups. Various media can be utilised, including interactive websites, electronic fact sheets/pamphlets, or videos.

One example is *InsideRadiology*, developed for the Australasian market in conjunction with the Royal Australian and New Zealand College of Radiologists (RANZCR).[24] This resource was developed by specialist radiologists and other content matter experts and then peer-reviewed by an editorial panel before publication. In addition to providing information regarding specific imaging modalities and tests, consumers are also offered general information regarding radiation safety, risks and benefits of imaging investigations and procedures and general information about radiology as a specialty within medicine.

Inclusive patient resources

Patients attending radiology services are diverse. Differences are encountered across ethnicity, culture, language, sexuality, gender identity and ability/disability. All patients are entitled to receive the highest quality of patient care. To achieve this, resources developed by radiology departments need to consider the diversity of the population they serve. Resources available to patients should be available for:

- A variety of languages and cultures, including those purposely developed for Indigenous peoples
- Hearing and visual impairment
- Different levels of health literacy and education

LGBTQIA+ populations have faced ongoing healthcare inequity and often have unique healthcare and psychological safety needs. Transgender patients, in particular, experience a disproportionate rate of harassment when engaging with medical services and too often have to educate their clinicians about how their gender identity impacts medical care.[25] It is important to consider gender identity and inclusiveness in providing department resources and creating signage. This includes the use of respectful communication (including gender-inclusive language) and reconsidering how gender terminology is used to describe medical imaging investigations. For example, the term 'women's imaging' reflects a lack of inclusivity for non-binary or transmasculine patients.[25] Inclusive language is also an important consideration in admissions processes (e.g. providing inclusive options for the nomination of sex or gender beyond a binary 'male or female'), and in direct patient-facing interactions.

BOX 1.9   PRACTICE QUESTIONS

- A patient has been booked for a CT-guided liver biopsy, and she asks if there is further information available for her to read prior to her procedure. How would you direct her?
- You have been asked to provide input to the design of a new patient information pamphlet for your medical imaging department. How could you make the resource more inclusive for the patient population?

CHALLENGES IN PATIENT COMMUNICATION

Breaking bad news

It is a misconception that radiologists do not have to be the bearers of 'bad news' to our patients. These scenarios most commonly arise during procedures and investigations where the medical imaging doctor is called upon to review a patient's scan in real time or is physically performing the investigation or procedure. One such heart-wrenching example is when a doctor is called by a sonographer to review an obstetric scan, and the foetal heartbeat is not present. Findings such as these require open and honest disclosure and are understandably fraught with emotion.

When breaking bad news to patients, it is important always to approach the conversation with empathy and compassion. A private and quiet environment is ideal. Clinicians should be honest and direct with the patient and those there to support them. The result or outcome should be explained in accessible language without medical jargon so that the patient should be able to comprehend the message regardless of their education status or health literacy.[23]

Breaking bad news can be emotionally taxing for the clinician and other medical imaging staff (such as radiographers and sonographers) involved in the patient's care. It is normal to be affected by such things. If needed, those involved should be offered a chance to debrief with supervisors or colleagues informally or formally, with the optional availability of formal psychological support services if required.

Communication errors

Communication errors are a leading cause of adverse events in medical imaging and healthcare settings. Just over one-third of communication errors in radiology were found to have a direct impact on patient care, with over half considered to have a potential impact.[26] Communication errors can occur at all stages of the clinician-patient interaction with medical imaging, including the time of study or procedure request, scheduling, performance, interpretation, and result communication. Disruption in communication can occur not only between staff members but also at the human-technology interface.

The electronic medical record reduces the risk of communication error by inbuilt checks and failsafe measures. Other strategies that can be used to reduce the risk of medication breakdown in the medical imaging department include the implementation of structured information transfer (for example, using the ISBAR[a] Handover mnemonic), developing and subsequent understanding of effective departmental/institutional policies, and incorporation of quality assurance measures.

Health literacy and communication mismatch

Communication can break down when a clinician cannot match the complexity of their language to the health literacy of the person they are interacting with (be they patient, family member or other support person). Medical staff possess a vast technical vocabulary, allowing them to communicate efficiently and proficiently in healthcare settings. Most patients, however, cannot follow the technicalities of medical conversation, leading to misunderstanding, frustration and disconnection – ultimately eroding the person-centred care model.

In direct patient interactions, the clinician must aim to explain the clinical concerns and important procedural information in a clear and accessible way, avoiding technical jargon. Communication can be iteratively adjusted through the consultation depending on interactive assessments of the patient's level of understanding. In addition, inviting the patient to ask questions and clarify key points (e.g. risks associated with a procedure) should be used to confirm understanding and build mutual respect.

Communicating with patients with limited fluency in English

The populations radiology departments serve are linguistically diverse, with some patients having limited proficiency in the English language. Patients with significant hearing impairment/deafness also encounter difficulties with conventional verbal communication. These barriers may not only lead to breakdowns in communication but also erode patient autonomy and result in disengagement with healthcare services.

Clear communication is paramount for all patients accessing medical imaging services to ensure safe and effective service delivery. This applies to both spoken communication and the provision of written support materials. Healthcare consumers who lack proficiency in English or are hearing impaired may require language support in the form of linguistically appropriate written materials and/or interpreter services.[27]

Patients who have limited fluency in English or who are deaf should be advised that they have the right to access interpreter services, and information should be provided in a timely fashion.[28] Ideally, this is in person; however, phone interpreters can be used in extenuating situations. Healthcare interpreters have undergone specialised training, are formally employed by the health service and are bound by professional codes of conduct. Family members or support persons fluent in the patient's preferred language should not act as interpreters, particularly in cases where informed consent is being sought, or there are significant implications for the patient's medical care.

When utilising interpreter services, communication should be clear and succinct but comprehensive. The clinician should pause after each sentence to allow the interpretation to take place. Where possible, pose questions directly to the patient to invite their response. Maintaining eye contact with the patient rather than the interpreter to build rapport and observe nonverbal cues is best.

Addressing radiation risk

In radiology and nuclear medicine, the small but real risks associated with radiation can lead to significant anxiety among patients. Community attitudes to radiation risk are widely varied, with some strong misconceptions about the dangers of radiation and radiation safety literacy often limited. This is balanced against increasing patient autonomy, with the patient-centred model of care championing that patients are well informed and encouraging them to participate actively in shared decision-making.

While consideration of radiation risk is important for all patients, particular care should be taken to adequately counsel patients who are potentially more vulnerable to the theoretical effects of radiation. This includes pregnant women and children.

It is more common for initial radiation safety counselling discussions to be between the patient and their referring clinician rather than between the radiologist and the patient. Difficulties can be encountered if the non-radiologist clinician has a limited understanding of radiobiology and cannot adequately and accurately address the patient's concerns regarding radiation risk. As such, it is important to encourage collaborative relationships between treating clinicians and local radiologists, which allow open discussion and a free line of communication to escalate questions. Radiologists should also be prepared to discuss radiation safety with patients under their care within the medical imaging department, particularly if the patient requests input from a medical doctor or the radiographers and other support staff cannot adequately address their concerns.

Radiation safety discussions can be difficult, particularly as the large body of knowledge is taken from extensive population-based studies that are not directly applicable to individuals. Strategies for broaching this conversation include:[29]

- Comparing the estimated radiation dose from the study to a common environmental exposure (e.g. a long-haul flight)
- Comparison of the mortality risk associated with radiation to the risks of common everyday behaviours (e.g. a short drive in a motor vehicle)
- Expressing additional cancer risk on top of background lifetime cancer risk

These strategies should be employed with care and tailored to each patient. It is not appropriate to advise the patient that there is "zero" risk of developing cancer with radiation, as a very small but theoretical risk exists. Conversely, it is important to avoid being alarmist in these discussions and keep the theoretical risks grounded within the context of the patient's care. Radiation safety counselling should always occur in conjunction with balancing the potential risk to the patient of not undergoing the test, i.e., the potential mortality and mobility of allowing the suspected condition to go undiagnosed/unmonitored.

Communicating with and managing anxious patients

Patients often attend medical imaging departments with heightened levels of anxiety related to the results of their upcoming diagnostic investigations, uncertainty of the process or apprehension in the face of an impending medical procedure. A feeling of anxiousness is a normal human response experienced by all people throughout their lives. This is distinct from an anxiety disorder, which is a mental health diagnosis.

Effective communication and information provision are key to helping patients feel less anxious. This starts before the patient arrives by ensuring they have been provided with clear information and instructions regarding their scan or procedure, understand why the test has been arranged, and are empowered to ask questions. Where possible, the information provided should be individualised.

For doctors consulting anxious patients in the department, communication must be clear and calm, allowing the patients to voice their concerns and answer questions. The clinicians should take the time to sympathise and empathise with the patient, that is, appreciating what the patient is feeling and also feeling it themself.[30] Radiologists need to be aware of their own emotional state and understand how this impacts patient interactions and care provision. The management of each anxious patient is unique and encompasses the individual patient's needs.

The patient should be encouraged to answer questions and seek clarification. Alternative management options (e.g. sedation) or alternative investigations can be discussed if clinically appropriate. Such conversations should occur through the lens of informed consent, with the cognisant of the knowledge they can revoke consent at any time.

Managing aggressive or violent patients

The manifestations of aggression and violence in healthcare settings are broad, encompassing a range of verbal and/or physical behaviours that occur with deliberate intent to threaten or cause harm. Physical violence can occur against people or property, including slamming doors and destruction of medical equipment. Aggressive and violent behaviour may manifest in patients or their support persons (e.g. relatives and friends).

Aggressive and violent behaviour is unfortunately encountered across healthcare settings, although it is less frequent in medical imaging departments compared to direct patient assessment settings such as the emergency department. Often, patients have been stabilised before their transport to the medical imaging department and screened for compliance with the investigation before arrival. Members of the medical imaging team, especially radiographers and sonographers, are at greater risk of confronting aggressive or violent persons as they are not only in more frequent direct contact with the patients but also routinely perform scans in mobile settings, e.g. emergency department, intensive care unit.

Medical imaging doctors may be called to speak with or review a patient or speak with a support person who is distressed, angry, or threatening violence. Their role is to assist with counselling the patient, de-escalating the situation, and/or providing support and assistance to other radiology team members. The clinician should attend the event in person if they are able and it is safe to do so.

Patients may be predisposed to aggression or violence as a manifestation of an underlying mental health or medical condition, including those that relate to the clinical presentation, such as delirium. The unfamiliar hospital environment, a sense of vulnerability and the fear and uncertainty around their acute illness can also exacerbate predispositions for aggression and violence.

TABLE 1.2   Management of the aggressive or violent patient.

PRE-EVENT	DURING THE EVENT	POST-EVENT
Creation of policies & procedures	Action as per policies & procedures	Documentation & incident reporting
Education and training including communication, de-escalation & conflict resolution skills	Activating alarms	Feedback/communication with managers & team
Risk assessments	Calling for help	Counselling & psychological support for involved/ affected staff
Installation & maintenance of warning systems and duress alarms	Removing staff & other patients from immediate danger	Review of systems & procedures
Removal of potential weapons from a space	De-escalation strategies	
Raise awareness of risks, policies & educational resources	Communication with imaging department staff, security & referring clinicians	

Adapted from Adeniyi & Puzi.[31]

The goals of managing aggressive or violent behaviour include ensuring staff safety and preventing the further escalation of the situation which could result in further harm. Assessment of the underlying condition is a secondary consideration; however, the imaging investigation required for this assessment should only proceed if it is safe for the staff and patient to do so.

Practical management of aggression and violence occurs before, during and after the event (Table 1.2).

When interacting with a distressed or aggressive person during the event, the clinician must remain calm and speak confidently and clearly. They should directly state that the behaviour is inappropriate and that compromises or bargains will not be made. Clear boundaries and limits should be set. However, it is equally important not to challenge the patient verbally or physically touch them. Staff should not turn their back on the aggressive person or make direct eye contact.[31]

Once the encounter has concluded, it should be discussed with the supervising staff and communicated to the managing clinical team (if they have not already been informed). Additional debriefing is often required to ensure the psychological safety of the staff involved and review the efficacy of policies and procedures in managing the situation.

BOX 1.10   PRACTICE QUESTIONS

- A radiographer comes to you for advice. A patient's referral requests a CT chest; however, the patient believes they have come for a CT abdomen and pelvis. How would you approach this?
- A patient has inadvertently had a CT of their brain instead of a CT of their head and neck. How would you approach communicating the error to the patient?

- What are three strategies that a radiologist could employ to assist in managing an anxious patient?
- The CT radiographer comes to you asking for assistance with an anxious patient who does not speak English. The contrast consent and screening questionnaire has not been completed. How would you approach this?
- A patient's mother asks you whether the CT brain study for her 3-year-old son could cause cancer. How would you respond to this?
- A patient has become verbally aggressive during a diagnostic ultrasound study. The sonographer calls you for help. How would you approach this scenario?

NOTE

a ISBAR: mnemonic used to guide structured communication in clinical handover. Introduce and identify, situation, background, assessment and actions, recommendations, requests or review.

REFERENCES

1. Mahnken AH, Boullosa Seoane E, Cannavale A, et al. CIRSE clinical practice manual. *CardioVascular and Interventional Radiology* 2021; *44*: 1323–1353.
2. Dutruel SP, Hentel KD, Hecht EM, et al. Patient-centered radiology communications: Engaging patients as partners. *Journal of the American College of Radiology*. Epub ahead of print 1 January 2023. DOI: 10.1016/j.jacr.2023.10.009
3. English W, Gott M, Robinson J. The meaning of rapport for patients, families, and healthcare professionals: A scoping review. *Patient Education and Counseling* 2022; *105*: 2–14.
4. Rasiah S, Jaafar S, Yusof S, et al. A study of the nature and level of trust between patients and healthcare providers, its dimensions and determinants: A scoping review protocol. *BMJ Open 10*. Epub ahead of print 23 January 2020. DOI: 10.1136/bmjopen-2018-028061
5. Australian Commission on Safety and Quality in Health Care. Person-centred care. *Australian Commission on Safety and Quality in Health Care*, https://www.safet yandquality.gov.au/our-work/partnering-consumers/person-centred-care (2023, accessed 26 April 2024).
6. Itri J. Patient-centered radiology. *Radiographics* 2015; *35*: 1835–1846.
7. Gallo A. What Is Active Listening? *Harvard Business Review*, 2024, https://hbr.org/2024/01/what-is-active-listening (2024, accessed 27 April 2024).
8. Abrahams R, Groysberg B. How to Become a Better Listener. *Harvard Business Review*, 2021, https://hbr.org/2021/12/how-to-become-a-better-listener (2021, accessed 27 April 2024).
9. Australian Commission on Safety and Quality in Healthcare. *Informed consent*, https://www.safetyandquality.gov.au/our-work/partnering-consumers/informed-consent (2024, accessed 29 April 2024).

10. New South Wales. Ministry of Health, NSW Health. *Consent to medical and healthcare treatment manual*. St Leonards, February 2020.
11. Royal Australian and New Zealand College of Radiologists. *Medical Imaging Informed Consent Guidelines*. Sydney, www.ranzcr.edu.au (2019).
12. Oseni AO, Chun J-Y, Morgan R, et al. Dealing with complications in interventional radiology. *CVIR Endovascular* 2024; 7: 32.
13. NSW Government. *Open Disclosure: Policy Directive*. Sydney, https://www1.health.nsw.gov.au/pds/ActivePDSDocuments/PD2023_034.pdf (18 October 2023, accessed 17 September 2024).
14. Hartung MP, Bickle IC, Gaillard F, et al. How to create a great radiology report. *Radiographics* 2020; 40: 1658–1670.
15. Busby LP, Courtier JL, Glastonbury CM. Bias in radiology: The how and why of misses and misinterpretations. *Radiographics* 2018; 38: 236–247.
16. Drew T, Võ ML-H, Wolfe JM. The invisible gorilla strikes again: Sustained inattentional blindness in expert observers. *Psychological Science* 2013; 24: 1848–1853.
17. Goodman LR. *Felson's Principles of Chest Roentgenology, A Programmed Text*. Elsevier Health Sciences, 2014.
18. Drew T, Võ ML-H, Olwal A, et al. Scanners and drillers: Characterizing expert visual search through volumetric images. *Journal of Visualization* 2013; 13: 3.
19. Turkbey B, Rosenkrantz AB, Haider MA, et al. Prostate imaging reporting and data system version 2.1: 2019 update of prostate imaging reporting and data system version 2. *European Urology* 2019; 76: 340–351.
20. Tessler FN, Middleton WD, Grant EG, et al. ACR thyroid imaging, reporting and data system (TI-RADS): White paper of the ACR TI-RADS committee. *Journal of the American College of Radiology* 2017; 14: 587–595.
21. Pool FJ, Ferris N, Siwach P, et al. Structured reporting in radiology: What do radiologists think and does RANZCR have a role in implementation. *Journal of Medical Imaging and Radiation Oncology* 2022; 66: 193–201.
22. Panicek DM, Hricak H. How sure are you, doctor? A standardized lexicon to describe the radiologist's level of certainty. *American Journal of Roentgenology* 2016; 207: 2–3.
23. Rockall AG, Justich C, Helbich T, et al. Patient communication in radiology: Moving up the agenda. *European Journal of Radiology* 155. Epub ahead of print 1 October 2022. DOI: 10.1016/j.ejrad.2022.110464
24. Royal Australian and New Zealand College of Radiologists (RANZCR). Inside Radiology. *RANZCR*, https://www.insideradiology.com.au/ (2019, accessed 16 September 2024).
25. Yan TD, Mak LE, Carroll EF, et al. Gender-inclusive fellowship naming and equity, diversity, and inclusion in radiology: An analysis of radiology department websites in Canada and the United States. *Canadian Association of Radiologists Journal* 2022; 73: 473–477.
26. Siewert B, Brook OR, Hochman M, et al. Impact of communication errors in radiology on patient care, customer satisfaction, and work-flow efficiency. *American Journal of Roentgenology* 2016; 206: 573–579.
27. NSW Health. *NSW Plan for Healthy Culturally and Linguistically Diverse Communities: 2019–2023*. Sydney, 6 May 2019.
28. NSW Health. NSW Health Care Interpreting Services, https://www.health.nsw.gov.au/multicultural/Pages/health-care-interpreting-and-translating-services.aspx (2024, accessed 17 September 2024).
29. Shyu JY, Sodickson AD. Communicating radiation risk to patients and referring physicians in the emergency department setting. *British Journal of Radiology* 2016; 89(1061): 20150868. Epub ahead of print 2016. DOI: 10.1259/bjr.20150868

30. Martinez Lorca A, Aguado Romo R, Martinez Lorca M, et al. Anxiety reduction and emotional self-care using the U-technique in radiology departments. *British Journal of Radiology* 2017; *90*: 20170173.
31. Adeniyi OV, Puzi N. Management approach of patients with violent and aggressive behaviour in a district hospital setting in South Africa. *South African Family Practice* 2021; *63*(4): 1–7.

Collaborating with Colleagues

2

DIVERSITY, EQUITY AND INCLUSION

The principles of diversity, equity, and inclusion permeate modern conversations around professional practice in radiology, and it is worthwhile to take some time to understand the definitions and impacts as we begin to discuss teamwork, collaboration, and department culture. Diversity, equity, inclusion, and how we uphold these in radiological practice will continue as a thread across upcoming chapters, especially as we review responsible practice, leadership, and medical imaging ethics.

Defining diversity, equity and inclusion

The **diversity** of a group considers the variation among its members and the differences between them. These differences can include (but are not limited to):[1]

- Gender, sex and sexual orientation
- Race, ethnicity, culture and religious/ethical beliefs
- Whether someone is differently abled or neurodivergent
- Social, financial and geographical status and upbringing
- Age

An organisation committed to diversity aims to acknowledge, respect, value and utilise the differences that people bring to a group rather than eliminate the differences between individuals.[2]

Equality considers all individuals equal and should be treated the same. While **equity** is similar, it also considers that some individuals have inherent disadvantages compared to others due to no fault of their own. Equity aims to account for these differences and essentially 'level the playing field'.

Inclusion combines the principles of diversity and equity. For example, a workplace may have a diverse staff across gender and ethnicity. Still, unless the differing perspectives of these team members are valued and respected in practice, the workplace would not be considered inclusive. Inclusive workplace practices are linked with greater

DOI: 10.1201/9781003466529-2

innovation, higher patient and customer satisfaction rates, improved mental health among employees and higher levels of job satisfaction.[3]

Diversity in radiology

Increased team diversity has been shown to have a range of benefits across different professional sectors, including healthcare. Diverse teams have been linked to improved employee and organisational performance, innovation and creativity, employee retention, greater engagement and positive impacts on well-being.[3, 4] These positive links translate into improved patient care delivery and better outcomes across healthcare teams, including medical imaging.

Diversity in the radiologist workforce has been a growing topic of conversation, particularly regarding the gender diversity of radiologists and training radiologists and the representation of minorities and First Peoples. In 2023, 30% of Australian radiologists and 31% of trainees were women, and 36% of New Zealand radiologists and 35% of trainees were women.[1] The gender discrepancy in training radiologists continues despite most medical schools in Australia and New Zealand graduating student cohorts at or near gender parity for decades. Australian and New Zealand data is similar to radiologist workforce diversity data from elsewhere around the world, where approximately one-third of the radiology workforce is made up of women.[5]

In the USA, demographic data also finds that there is an underrepresentation of some ethnicities (including African American or Hispanic people) across radiology practice, with the lack of diversity more pronounced at senior academic and leadership levels.[6]

Chapter 5 explores different forms of diversity and strategies for making patient care and workplaces more inclusive in more detail.

Intersectionality

Intersectionality considers the impact of overlapping forms of disadvantage and/or discrimination based on a person's identity. Understanding this principle is important in designing and implementing any strategies targeting diversity or inequity, as plans targeting a single diversity metric can have significant inadvertent consequences for other minority groups. For example, a review of academic radiologist salaries comparing intersectional groups in the USA found that in interventional radiology faculties, Asian women had the greatest pay discrepancy – earning 15% less than white men of the same rank.[7]

Allyship and pronouns

The Pride Network at the University of Sydney provides a comprehensive definition of allyship:

An ally encompasses anyone, irrespective of their sexual orientation, gender identity, or sex characteristics, who actively advocates for LGBTQIA+ inclusion. The fundamental role of an ally is to remain informed about the obstacles encountered by LGBTQIA+ individuals and to contribute to positive change. This may entail serving as a supportive contact or taking a stand against any form of inequity or exclusion. An ally is furthermore a catalyst for transformation, actively confronting and countering homophobia, transphobia, biphobia, heterosexism, and interphobia.[8]

For practising radiologists, understanding allyship and constantly reflecting on your behaviour and those of others is essential. This extends across the medical imaging department as a workplace into interactions with patients, who should feel safe and respected while engaging with medical imaging services.

Gender pronouns (e.g. he/him, she/her, they/them) denote the preferred way an individual would like to be described, reflecting their gender identity. Gender and sex are not interchangeable. A person's sex reflects the biological and physical characteristics of males and females, whereas gender exists as a spectrum that encompasses complex psychosocial self-perceptions and external expectations.[4]

The choice of whether to disclose one's gender pronouns lies with the individual. Disclosure should not be mandated or forced by a department or organisation. If an individual feels safe to do so, sharing pronouns in conversation or electronic communication can help signal safety and promote inclusive workplace practices. This is equally, if not more, important for cis-gendered individuals. Using the correct pronouns for a coworker or patient shows basic respect and validation.

BOX 2.1   PRACTICE QUESTIONS

- Define diversity and equity as they relate to the clinical radiology workforce.
- Describe some ways in which a diverse radiology workforce can positively impact workplace culture and patient care.

PRINCIPLES FOR WORKING WITHIN MEDICAL IMAGING AND WIDER HEALTHCARE TEAMS

The success of the healthcare team is paramount to providing high-quality patient care. Well-functioning teams have the potential to navigate complex healthcare challenges better, reduce medical errors and adverse outcomes, increase job satisfaction, and improve the health and well-being of team members.[9] The diagnostic and procedural radiology process represents a partnership between the medical imaging and referring teams, meaning that communication breakdowns can potentially harm patients if they are not recognised and effectively managed.

Radiology in the diagnostic process[10]

The diagnostic process models the steps a patient moves through as they are managed for a health problem, recognising that clinicians must adequately understand the patient's condition to determine the best management course. Steps in the diagnostic process are summarised in Figure 2.1.

The diagnostic process model simplifies the complexities of patient care in many cases, and its success is determined by the accuracy of the examinations and tests and the skills of the clinicians involved in interpretation and clinical problem-solving.

Diagnostic imaging is typically involved early in the diagnostic process, with additional examinations undertaken or studies repeated over the patient's journey. Radiologists plays an important role in the initial refinement of the working diagnosis and subsequent monitoring and/or re-evaluation, specifically:

- Determining the appropriateness of medical imaging tests to answer the clinical question or corroborate the working diagnosis
- Deciding on the most appropriate imaging modality and study protocol
- Interpretation of the test and integration of imaging findings with other clinical information

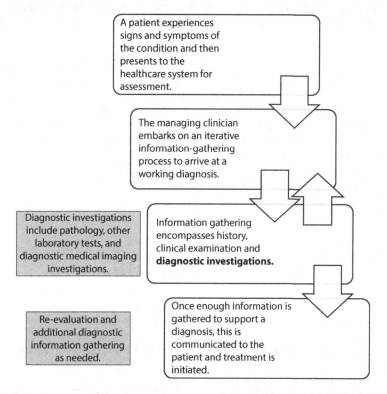

FIGURE 2.1   Summary of the diagnostic process. Adapted from Larson & Langlotz.[10]

Additionally, interventional radiology can be involved in the diagnostic process to gather information or at the treatment stage.

The success of the diagnostic process requires clear communication between the managing clinicians and the radiology teams. This includes, but is not limited to, the provision of adequate but succinct information in imaging referrals, the creation of clear imaging reports and participation in multidisciplinary discussions (see *Chapter 1: The Written Radiology Report* and *Chapter 2: Imaging Professionals in Multidisciplinary Teams*).

Teamwork in medical imaging departments

Factors that can influence the quality of the medical imaging team (or any healthcare professional team) can be divided into general teamwork, emotional climate, patient safety, and education (Table 2.1). As a large team and/or organisation dynamic is complex and changeable, many factors can overlap or influence each other. For example, suppose a radiology trainee does not clearly understand the scope of their daily clinical responsibilities. In that case, there is the potential for breakdowns in communication, escalating stress and fatigue, and ultimately impacting the quality of patient care by causing delays in arranging or reporting scans or resulting in medical error.

In imaging, a team may be as small as a few clinicians working together on a research project or as big as an entire medical imaging department in a large tertiary

TABLE 2.1   Factors influencing teamwork in medical imaging practice.

TEAMWORK GENERAL FACTORS	*EMOTIONAL CLIMATE FACTORS*
• Defined roles & responsibilities • Shared identity & commitment • Interdependence between members • Integrative & collaborative work practices • Effective communication • Engagement, positive feedback & recognition • Adequate staffing • Authentic leadership • Diverse team composition • Adaptability to change	• Stress & fatigue • Team building & wellness activities • Perceptions of team members • Psychological safety • Inclusive workplace practices • Disruptive behaviours
PATIENT SAFETY FACTORS	*EDUCATION FACTORS*
• Healthcare fragmentation • Authority imbalance • Lack of coordination • Communication tools • Patient safety training/skills • Distractions, interruptions & disruptions • Accountability processes	• Interprofessional workshops • Simulation • Teamwork-specific activities • Continuing professional education • Involvement in education & training

Adapted from Parra et al.[9]

healthcare centre. While the specifics of what makes an effective team can vary greatly, successful collaborations often have key characteristics in common:[11]

- Meaningful **common purpose(s)** the team takes ownership of, which is appropriate and realistic e.g. high-quality patient care, excellent quality of medical images and reports, world-class delivery of procedural radiology services
- Specific **performance goals** that flow from the common purpose e.g. timely performance and interpretation of diagnostic imaging, improved waiting times for access to interventional procedures
- A mix of **complementary and diverse skills** among team members
- A solid **commitment** for completion of work, as part of the daily practice necessities and broader long-term projects
- Mutual **accountability** between all team members, including the leader/s

Medical imaging departmental culture

The culture of a team, department or organisation provides the foundation for the work that is done and the outcomes that are produced. Culture is a complex social and professional construct but could be likened to the 'personality' of the department or organisation.[12] It is the way people collectively behave and the attitudes and beliefs which shape those behaviours.[12] Determinates of culture include:[13]

- Observable practices (actions and behaviours)
- Values of individual team members and the organisation
- Fundamental assumptions including conscious and unconscious perceptions and biases, and feelings towards these

People from various professions work together in the medical imaging department to deliver high-quality patient care. This includes doctors, radiographers, sonographers and other imaging technologists, nurses, administrators, patient support officers, and students. A professional group comprises people with different skillsets, training levels, and responsibilities. For example, 'doctors' within the medical imaging department may include specialists, trainees/residents, junior medical staff and medical students. Even specialists and trainees will span disciplines such as diagnostic and interventional radiology, nuclear medicine and other specialties e.g. cardiologists who interpret CT coronary angiography or cardiac MRI. The health of these inter- and intra-professional relationships shapes the department's culture.

A workplace's culture can potentially impact its members for better or worse. Positive workplace cultures can benefit workers' mental health and well-being, improve job satisfaction, promote employee retention and deliver better-quality patient care.

What constitutes a 'good' culture of radiology is challenging to define. What constitutes a good culture in medical imaging will vary across healthcare settings and geography; however, some considerations include:[14]

- Acceptable balance of diagnostic and procedural workload demands and resources/time allocated
- A sense of community and connection
- Inclusive workplace practices (i.e. fostering a sense of belonging)
- Psychologically safe behaviours and just culture
- Cultural, social and gender diversity
- Creativity and innovation
- A sense of genuine appreciation and value

Accountability and self-awareness

Our success as a team member is not solely reliant on our ability to navigate the heterogeneity of personalities, skills and attitudes of those we work with. Instead, it should be driven by an awareness of our own personal and professional behaviours, attitudes and biases before all else. This includes reflecting on one's:[15]

- Internal self-awareness
- External self-awareness
- Personal accountability

Internal self-awareness holds that if we have a better understanding of our own emotions, assumptions and biases, we not only have a better understanding of the behaviours and actions of others but are less likely to make excuses for our own conduct.

BOX 2.2   FOR EXAMPLE …

Consider a case of a missed clinically significant finding in a CT study. If it was a colleague, a team member with a lack of internal self-awareness might be quick to judge the error as resulting from a lack of skill or negligence. If it was their error, they may be quick to downplay the mistake due to the complexity of the case or a roster that was too demanding.

In contrast, **external self-awareness** recognises how our actions impact the behaviour of those around us. This is particularly important for leaders and team members in positions of authority. External self-awareness can be a humbling skill to hone and develop, particularly as we may not like the perceptions that others hold about us. Gaining a sense of the attitudes of others to us can be achieved by observing other team members or seeking direct, honest feedback (which can be a confronting exercise).

Personal accountability considers the findings and reflections of internal and external self-awareness and grows beyond this into action and change. Should a problem with our own conduct arise, whether it be personal or arising as part of the team's business, the member with strong personal accountability identifies and accepts the problem meaningfully. They then go on to personally take responsibility for the issue and engage in concrete steps to address it – persisting until a resolution is met.

Psychological safety

Psychological safety is the " 'perception that an environment is safe for interpersonal risk-taking, exposing vulnerability, and contributing perspectives without fear of being shamed, blamed or ignored.'[16] Psychologically safe professional environments correlate with high-quality patient care, innovative practices and a greater sense of meaning and belonging among employees. In comparison, workplaces not considered to be psychologically safe risk detriment to the mental health and the well-being of team members, and are linked to poorer outcomes for patients. The growth and innovation within a department may also be stunted by the reluctance of staff to vocalise ideas, take calculated risks, and/or maintain accountability for perceived errors.

The radiology learning space has inherent challenges in establishing psychological safety, including:[17]

* Hierarchical professional relationships
* Established educational practices such as live case readouts, case conferences and 'hot seat'-style tutorials
* The apprenticeship model where training radiologists learn by having their work consistently corrected and reviewed.

Such educational practices may inadvertently evoke excessive stress, embarrassment or shame within learners if they are not conducted with care.

Psychological safety in a radiology department can be improved by:[18]

* Building professional and educational relationships
* Setting realistic and meaningful expectations
* Promoting a culture valuing inclusivity and openness
* Maintaining a primary focus on patient care

The challenge of learning radiology to obtain a fellowship requires a degree of commitment and accountability on the part of the training doctor. A certain degree of pressure is necessary to drive engagement with, and retention of, the high level of knowledge expected of a qualified radiologist. This necessary stress must be balanced against maintaining a psychologically safe environment where learners can make mistakes and grow from the lessons learned.

Emotional intelligence, trust and loyalty in teams

Broadly, **emotional intelligence** is the measure of an individual's ability to manage themselves and others, with five core components:[19]

- Self-awareness
- Self-regulation
- Motivation
- Empathy
- Social skills

Emotional intelligence predicts doctor well-being, positively impacting stress management for the individual doctor, reducing burnout and improving engagement with education and training. Higher emotional intelligence is also linked to better-quality doctor–patient interactions, empathy, teamwork, communication skills, organisational commitment and leadership.[20] Emotional intelligence is a skill that can be developed over time by the individual (e.g. through self-reflection, active listening and seeking and responding to feedback), or through formal training (e.g. unconscious bias training, leadership or teamwork development workshops).

Establishing trust in teams is built on mutual respect, ideally forged by shared commitments and values within a team or broader organisation. Trust cannot be forced or coerced, and it is not a given that individuals trust those in leadership positions.

Loyalty is the emotional commitment to a team or organisation, manifesting as engagement with common goals and practical work. It reflects the value that a person feels they hold and contribute. If this sense is absent, the individual may feel stressed, angry, disengaged, or apathetic, risking employee health and eventual resignation.

Leaders can foster loyalty within their organisation; however, like trust, they cannot coerce or force it. Loyalty can be encouraged if leaders exercise empathy and compassion, demonstrate a genuine interest and understanding of the ideas and perspectives of others and act with authenticity and assertiveness.[21]

Defining roles and responsibilities

The quality of teamwork and collaboration is enhanced when individuals are given a clear indication of their roles, responsibilities and expectations. It was previously believed that leaving the definitions of roles open would encourage creativity and flexibility; however, the opposite was found to be true.[22] Team members need to clearly understand what is within and outside the scope of their work and the complementary scope of others they collaborate with. These individuals work within their defined parameters towards a common goal – be that something overarching, such as the delivery of patient care, or something specific, such as completing a department-wide audit of CT pulmonary angiograms.

The leader, whether a clinical director, section or group chief, or project manager, is responsible for defining team members' roles. The leader also has the prerogative to ensure that the team members they collaborate with clearly understand individual goals and expectations. Team members should be allowed to discuss the suitability of these, and suggest changes for consideration.

This said, the definition of an individual's scope of work is not a checklist exercise, and room to exercise autonomy, flexibility and creativity within the broad guidelines is essential. Strategies to improve this include:[23]

- Recognising excellence and rewarding it tangibly (on both small and larger scales)

- Setting motivating goals which are realistically achievable and guided by time frames
- Letting people decide the specifics of 'how' they work towards the prescribed goals (within organisational expectations and limitations)

BOX 2.3   PRACTICE QUESTIONS

- Outline some factors that may impact the teamwork dynamic in a medical imaging department. Give an example of how a breakdown in teamwork can impact radiology service delivery and patient care.
- You have been asked to report an urgent prostate MRI, but do not feel you have adequate expertise in this area. How would you approach this?
- Define psychological safety, and explain its importance in educating medical imaging registrars/residents.

MANAGING COMMUNICATION BREAKDOWNS AND CONFLICT

Conflict in the workplace is a highly undesirable, but often inevitable part of professional practice. In these situations, it can be difficult to think clearly or act in the ideal capacity according to our values or those of the organisation. Conflict escalating between colleagues can create a challenging work environment. It has the potential to impact the health and well-being of the individual, broader team and patients, with a North American study finding that a quarter of hospital staff feeling that disruptive behaviour had played a part in the death of a patient.[24] As such, it is important to approach conflict or potential conflict with open dialogue, humility, and a desire to reach a satisfactory outcome that aligns with the principles of practice.

Defining interpersonal conflict

Interpersonal conflict occurs between individuals where adverse emotional reactions occur secondary to perceived disagreement or interference with goals, aspirations or tasks.[25] It is a dynamic process encompassing different levels and severities of negative interactions and intent to harm.

Examples of negative behaviours that can manifest in interpersonal conflict include:[26]

- **Defensiveness:** deflection of critical feedback elsewhere, e.g. onto a colleague or the organisation
- **Victim mentality:** perception of being unfairly singled out, targeted or held to a higher standard compared to other colleagues

- **Passive aggressiveness:** indirect resistance to requests and avoidance of direct discussion or confrontation
- **Bullying:** deliberate and repeated behaviours aimed at an individual with the intent to cause harm or intimidation
- **Vertical aggression:** bullying behaviours directed at leaders (usually new leaders) by experienced or strongly opined staff members
- **Informant:** staff communicating concerns to managers and leaders about the conduct of their colleague without objective evidence

Bullying[27]

Workplace bullying has unfortunately been found to be overrepresented in healthcare settings and, as such, is a problem encountered in medical imaging departments. While there is no universally agreed definition of bullying, the behaviours are usually repetitive and performed with the intent to cause harm or distress. The behaviour can be physical, verbal or psychological and include abuse, humiliation, intimidation and insults severe enough to impact individual work performance. Bullying can occur between individuals or groups and span face-to-face and online interactions.

Victims may experience a range of negative impacts, including:

- Loss of self-confidence
- Embarrassment
- Vulnerability
- Psychological stress and distress
- Detrimental effects to physical and mental health

Patients can be negatively impacted, particularly in circumstances of long-term bullying, as clinicians become less engaged with their work and lose confidence. Bullying can also lead to a lack of focus, raising the risk of medical errors. There is the potential to negatively impact future generations of doctors and radiologists, particularly if they witness the modelling of bullying behaviour by senior clinicians or are impacted by the loss of confidence and engagement suffered by the victims.

Feedback processes, review, and education by intellectual challenge or questioning (Socratic Method) are not considered bullying behaviours but rather an important part of continuing education and quality improvement. Should Socratic teaching methods degrade into a situation where direct harm is caused to the learner, this can develop into bullying behaviour.

The medical imaging department leadership is responsible for addressing these behaviours in the workplace, with most departments and broader healthcare organisations having a specific code of conduct in place. This includes providing specific definitions of what constitutes bullying and workplace disruption and outlines the obligations staff have regarding their own behaviour and duty of care to report such behaviours if they are witnessed.

If bullying behaviour is witnessed, this should be discussed with a supervisor. For a radiology trainee, the first port of call is usually the director of radiology training/ program director.

Disruptive behaviour

The spectrum of disruptive behaviour in a workplace encompasses a range of unprofessional behaviours which vary in severity and intent. Broadly, these behaviours are misaligned with the healthcare/medical imaging team's goals and can degrade departmental culture, interpersonal relationships and patient care. In addition, persistent disruptive behaviours have been linked to increased rates of medical errors and escalating healthcare delivery costs.[28]

Disruptive behaviours may present as aggressive or overt actions, for example, verbal or physical abuse, sexual or other forms of harassment, threats or bullying, or more intermediate but still damaging actions such as hoarding of information, engaging in gossip or devaluation of the time or contribution of team members.

Devaluation can manifest as chronic lateness, sarcastic comments, exclusionary behaviour, continued checking of mobile devices during times of expected focus or carrying out private conversations during teaching sessions or meetings.[13] Microaggressions and passive-aggressive behaviour are also considered disruptive behaviours. Disruptive behaviours can overlap with mental health conditions and substance use disorders (which impact approximately 10–12% of healthcare professionals).[28]

For radiology trainees engaging in formalised apprenticeship learning, demonstrating disruptive behaviours during educational activities can erode the integrity of the educational experience and risk alienating the teacher. Given the inherent reliance on the goodwill of senior medical staff to educate within the specialty training pathway, disruptive behaviours could fracture the quality and volume of radiology education available to trainees.

In contrast, should a more senior member of the medical team exhibit behaviours that devalue the educational or professional activity, it can erode the academic engagement of other learners – especially training radiologists.[28] Examples include routine lateness or early departure, falling asleep during presentations or clinical work, or preoccupation with phones or other electronic devices.

Triggers of disruptive behaviours[13]

A range of factors over short or longer periods can trigger disruptive behaviour. The types of triggers can be broadly divided into three groups:

- Intrapersonal triggers
- Interpersonal triggers
- Situational triggers

Intrapersonal triggers are unique to each person's context and are contained within the individual. These encompass one's culture, beliefs, perceptions, conscious and unconscious biases, and professional competence and confidence. Intrapersonal triggers that result in disruptive behaviour are more likely to manifest during times of crisis or when quick thinking or decision-making is required.

Interpersonal triggers encompass how the individual interacts with others in the professional environment. They are influenced by team dynamics, the diversity and inclusiveness of the work environment, leadership styles, and others' stereotypes.

Situational triggers may relate to the broader organisation or institution or the individual's personal and professional stressors. Organisational situational triggers include:

- Workplace culture
- Policies, procedures and systems
- The physical work environment

Situational triggers include staff members' perceptions of the organisation's values and actions. For example, if an organisation claims that patient care should be the highest priority, but staff perceive financial gain as more important, it can trigger disruption and conflict.

In addition to the triggers experienced in healthcare in general, there are additional specific challenges for medical imaging departments. The long-held stereotype of the money-driven and isolated radiologist, who avoids interactions with patients and other doctors can be damaging to both the individual and the group, with the potential to act as an intrapersonal or interpersonal trigger. Other examples include:

- Increasing reporting workloads
- Reporting list backlogs
- Financial pressures and performance indices (e.g. key performance indicators, measuring of revenue generation per scan reported)
- Changing/evolving imaging modalities, technologies and reporting requirements
- Technological/IT disruptions
- Competing/conflicting commitments (e.g. reporting duties competing with multidisciplinary team meeting preparation and attendance)
- Education commitments (i.e. training registrars/residents)
- Feedback and error reporting

Communication breakdown between medical staff

Patient harm can result from a breakdown in communication between radiologists and their colleagues, both within and outside the imaging department.

Radiology reports often include advice on managing urgent or incidental findings and recommendations for additional imaging. This creates inherent vulnerability should the results not be communicated clearly, promptly, or at all. Should a report require amendment, the radiologist is further obligated to ensure that clinically significant updates are directly conveyed to those responsible for the patient's care.

Often, the breakdown in communication itself is multifactorial and influenced by:

- Human interactions
- Technological factors (including electronic medical records and information sharing)
- Institutional practice, policy and culture

In radiology practice especially, safe communication of test results and procedural documentation between healthcare teams is particularly vulnerable. This risk is greatest when there is a transfer of care between clinicians and/or other healthcare providers and when reports are amended by the reporting radiologist.[29] The incidence of communication breakdown can be reduced by vigilance on behalf of the clinician with clear documentation and via the integration and appropriate use of electronic medical systems.

BOX 2.4   FOR EXAMPLE ...

Should radiologists identify clinically urgent findings or add an addendum to the report with new clinical implications, they should engage in direct discussion with the managing clinician. The nature of the interaction should be documented in the radiology report, including the names of the professionals contacted and the time and date when the handover took place.

Principles for managing conflict

As the manifestations of conflict within an imaging department can be broad, there is no one best way to mitigate and resolve such grievances. However, some common themes and trends among departmental culture and leadership styles are noted to be most conducive to effective conflict management. At the outset, it is important to remember that we and our colleagues are all humans who make mistakes and can, at times, act out of step with our personal values.

Collegial departmental culture and transformational and authoritative/aspirational leadership styles have been found to positively impact the conflict mitigation process, with authoritative and transactional styles having the potential to negate conflict resolution.[25] (see *Chapter 2: Medical Imaging Leadership Skills.*)

Any strategies employed by the organisation should be supported by evidence-based policies and guidelines, which ideally should be in place to resolve conflict before it arises. When determining strategies for managing conflict, factors to consider can be broadly categorised according to:[25]

- Individual characteristics
- Contextual factors
- Interpersonal conditions

When gauging the **individual characteristics** of those involved, it is important to consider their emotional intelligence, perceptions, attitudes, beliefs, and personality traits. These individual factors will be influenced by their demographics (including ethnicity, culture, and gender), motives, and experiences.

Broader **contextual factors** will be influenced by the departmental culture and work environment and by any policies and procedures regarding decision-making and resourcing. The clear definition of employee roles and responsibilities (or lack thereof) should be carefully considered, particularly if the conflict relates to tasks, aspirations or duties.

Interpersonal conditions include evaluating the relationship between the involved parties, including any communication breakdowns, erosion of trust, or perceived lack of support. Considering interpersonal conditions is important for understanding not only the context in which the conflict has arisen but also what barriers may exist to reaching a satisfactory resolution.

Specific interventions may relate to mediation processes, stress reduction initiatives, coaching or psychological interventions such as cognitive behaviour therapy. Furthermore, raising awareness and promoting education around the detection, acknowledgement and mitigation of disruptive behaviours and conflict amongst medical imaging department staff and leadership teams can help to prevent and better manage the situations should they arise.[25, 30]

Should a peaceful resolution not be possible, managers or staff may need to involve organisations or advocacy groups outside the medical imaging department. This could include medical indemnity organisations or employee/industry unions, who could be called upon to advise or represent individuals or groups of staff.

Personal communication in conflict

Conflict can bring out the worst in ourselves and our colleagues. Approaching interpersonal disagreement requires empathy, self-reflection and openness. Escalating disruptions and simmering conflicts are best managed with open and calm discussion, but how this is broached between individuals will vary.

Gallo suggests seven strategies that may help to open lines of communication and mitigate disruptions:[31]

1. Consider the viewpoints of others and remember that everyone has individual opinions, attitudes and biases
2. Be aware of your own unconscious biases
3. Avoid framing the conflict as 'me against them'
4. Have a clear vision of your priorities and goals before addressing the conflict
5. Check in with trusted coworkers, but be wary of damaging gossip and venting
6. Try different strategies to determine what works and what doesn't
7. Approach communications around conflict with an open mind and curiosity

Despite the best intentions of those involved, not all conflicts can be resolved peacefully or productively. In these cases, the issues should be escalated to a manager or supervisor, or discussed with the organisation's human resources department. Should the situation give rise to mental health and psychological stressors, staff should seek assistance from well-being support services.

BOX 2.5   PRACTICE QUESTIONS

- A junior doctor requests a CT pulmonary angiogram, firmly stating that they want the study performed without contrast. After you tell them it isn't possible they sternly tell you that you have to do the scan because their 'boss' wants it. How do you manage this?

• You witness a junior radiology colleague bullying another junior colleague on several occasions. How would you manage this scenario?

IMAGING PROFESSIONALS IN MULTIDISCIPLINARY TEAMS

Multidisciplinary patient management is paramount to comprehensive healthcare delivery, with medical imaging a crucial part of this team. The benefits of radiology involvement in multidisciplinary care are broad. However, the practical implications of facilitating this can pose challenges. Medical imaging services can be a part of multidisciplinary care in a broad sense as part of a wider healthcare service or fill a more specific role as a representative member of a multidisciplinary team (MDT) (or multidisciplinary team meeting [MDM]) managing the care needs of more complex patients.

Defining multidisciplinary care, teams and meetings

Multidisciplinary care is provided when multiple health professionals of different disciplines collaborate in the interest of one or more patients. Team composition is not limited to clinical doctors but can involve allied health staff (e.g., dietitians, physiotherapists, occupational therapists), nurses, and administrators involved in coordinating care. MDTs can exist across inpatient, outpatient and community healthcare settings, with the composition changing according to the priorities of care and practice setting.

The goal of the MDT is to provide the highest level of comprehensive care possible, which may vary over time as the needs of the patient(s) change. MDT discussion and collaboration has been shown to directly impact patient diagnosis, management and choice of investigations – improving diagnostic quality and certainty.[32] For some conditions, including interstitial lung disease, the gold standard for diagnosis is MDT discussion – rather than clinical findings alone or any diagnostic test.

Characteristics of an effective multidisciplinary team include:[33]

• Effective communication
• Efficient coordination
• Respect and trust between team members/disciplines
• Clear and robust implementation strategies
• Transparency in governance and decision-making practices

Other broad principles of effective teams will impact the success of the MDT (see *Chapter 2: Principles for Working within Medical Imaging and Wider Healthcare Teams*).

The MDM is a formal meeting where the MDT comes together to discuss specific patients with the aim of collaborative, shared decision-making in management decisions. It is now considered the standard of care for many patient groups with complex care needs, such as patients with cancer, recent stroke, or complex cardiovascular surgery. The chair of the MDM is usually a senior clinician.

The value of radiology in the multidisciplinary team

Radiologist and nuclear medicine specialist involvement is variable across MDTs and MDMs. Medical imaging representation offers greater value in teams with a core diagnostic imaging component in the cases presented and/or where interventional radiology expertise may be consulted. For example, in the Thoracic Oncology MDM, diagnostic radiology and PET/CT image presentation and review (by radiology and nuclear medicine specialists, respectively) is crucial to determining patient disease stage and suitability for specific lines of treatment. The presence of an interventional radiologist's opinion is highly valued for advice on the approach to biopsy of potential thoracic cancers or in managing treatment complications.

The benefits of involving radiology within the MDT/MDM can be divided into:

- Benefits for the patient
- Benefits for the radiologist
- Benefits for the broader healthcare community

For **patients**, there is value in having the opportunity to present and re-review pertinent imaging studies. By directly presenting and reviewing the images in real time, the clinicians directly involved in the care and decision-making for the patient can develop plans and seek second opinions from their colleagues in and outside of their specialty. Imaging studies can be re-reviewed (ideally by an imaging expert with a special interest in the presented conditions), increasing diagnostic accuracy. The added benefit is that the second review usually occurs in the setting of additional clinical information, investigation results, and the ability to seek clinical correlation in real time.

For the individual **radiologist**, participation in the MDT/MDM offers an opportunity to participate in a high-yield professional development activity, offering complex cases with clinical and radiology-pathology (rad-path) correlation and real-time feedback. By witnessing and participating in MDM discussions, radiologists are also allowed to learn more about novel therapies and emerging trends in patient care. On a personal level, the collaboration and connection the meeting offers can bring the radiologist a sense of value and purpose, as well as add interest and variation to their daily clinical practice.

Conversely, **other members of the MDT** are given the opportunity to learn from radiologists and nuclear medicine specialists. Radiologists and nuclear medicine specialists can impart knowledge of:

- Specific imaging findings and how they potentially impact management decisions

- Which imaging modalities and tests are most appropriate for investigation for different clinical questions and contexts
- The role interventional/procedural radiology can play in the diagnosis and treatment of complex conditions
- The potential benefits of collaborating with imaging teams in research and quality assurance initiatives

In a general sense, the willing participation of radiologists in the MDT is crucial for the visibility of the specialty.[34] By highlighting the availability and willingness of medical imaging representatives to collaborate across disciplines, there is greater opportunity for involvement in research, quality assurance and educational activities. With the establishment of strong professional relationships comes the added expectation that radiologists will be available and willing to speak on behalf of their specialty when healthcare policy and other broader projects are being discussed, and governance decisions are made.

Increasing the visibility of medical imaging has the added benefit of showcasing expert role models for medical students and junior staff who are also routinely in attendance at MDMs. Radiology and nuclear medicine can be seen as an aspirational and viable future career goal if presenters model the specialty as intellectually stimulating and showcase the benefits of radiology to the patient care journey.

Virtual and hybrid multidisciplinary meetings

During the COVID-19 pandemic, the availability of online and hybrid MDT meeting options sharply increased. In the years that have followed, many MDMs have adopted a hybrid approach (i.e., with some attendees physically present and others joining online) and others remain wholly online. The initial barriers of unfamiliarity with teleconferencing technology and the inherent quality of the platforms have improved with time.

The continued option to attend MDMs and other clinical meetings virtually has the benefit of improved flexibility for attendees and increased accessibility for those who may be otherwise prevented from participating by distance/geography, available time, or other competing commitments. For radiologists and others presenting clinical images, the option to project screens from clinical workstations/PACS systems has also been useful. The MDM benefits from these advantages – potentially improving the diversity and quality of expertise among attendees, enjoying the provision of high-quality images, and the ability to review comparative studies on the fly.

Challenges with online or hybrid meetings arise when communication and professional collaboration are hindered or broken down. Socially, online meetings separate the presenter and the audience, so both presenter and audience lose the sense of connection and real-time feedback gained by reading non-verbal cues. Audiences are also more likely to stay silent if online and are less likely to ask 'off-the-cuff' questions or chime in casual comments. Professional relationships that form organically with in-person meetings may be hindered or not develop if contact is wholly online, potentially impacting future interdisciplinary collaboration. While technology has improved, the potential impact of technical impairments or gaps in technology literacy can also represent an ongoing barrier to the success of online or hybrid meetings.

Strategies for leading an effective clinical meeting

Clinical meeting structure and organisation is variable. Large multidisciplinary team meetings in tertiary referral hospitals often bring representatives across clinical and diagnostic specialties, commonly with a nursing or administrative support person or team working behind the scenes to coordinate referrals and collect information in preparation for discussion. Smaller meetings may comprise doctors and other care coordinators in a single speciality, providing the radiologist with a list of patients where an imaging review would impact care decisions or represent an interesting learning opportunity.

Meeting leadership and record keeping

The meeting chairperson will be agreed upon in advance, often established by precedent. For example, in the head and neck cancer MDT meeting, the chair may be a head and neck surgeon in one centre and a radiation oncologist in another centre. For some meetings, particularly if imaging review is the focus, the radiologist may effectively drive the meeting – working through a patient list provided by the attendees. The chair's role is to moderate discussions, clarify the formal recommendation or diagnosis (if relevant) and keep the meeting moving forward so that all patients can be reviewed within the allocated time. The chair may scribe, or another staff member delegated minute-taking duties.

Preparation and image review

Before attending the clinical meeting, the medical imaging delegate should take the time to review each scan and compare their findings to those in the report. As the clinical meeting is part of the peer-review process, the imaging preparation should not be limited to correlating the conclusions described in the report. The review is an opportunity for an expert second opinion, which can be refined with additional clinical information, discussion and hindsight. If a radiology registrar/resident is preparing and/or presenting the meeting, this should be done under a specialist's close supervision and guidance.

Presenting cases to the MDM

When presenting the radiology images, it is customary for the team to provide the clinical history before launching into the case presentation. Descriptions should be succinct and focus on providing information that will impact decision-making. For example, when presenting a lung cancer case, it is important to describe the tumour's location, measure dimensions, describe the lesion's characteristics, and assess whether it is contacting or invading any local structures such as the pleura. This information is provided as it is needed to correctly assign a 'T' stage to the tumour – a grading that assists with management.

　　The presentation should focus on the condition under discussion or the specific question the referring team poses. Clinically significant incidental findings should be clearly stated at the end of the presentation to ensure the team is aware. Lengthy descriptions and repetition should be avoided in the interest of time and moving the meeting forward.

Presentations should be delivered clearly and steadily. Your speaking volume will vary depending on whether the meeting is delivered in person, over teleconference, or in a hybrid setting. It is best to avoid technical radiology jargon, keeping the presentation's lexicon pitched at the level of the general medical community. If technical descriptions or novel signs are part of the presentation, providing a 1–2-sentence explanation for the room may be pertinent to help others understand.

Displaying and showcasing images

With the wide availability of electronic PACS systems, MDT presentations are usually performed with interactive cases, scrollable in the case of cross-sectional imaging studies. The MDT presentation is a form of visual storytelling, and it is the role of the presenter to determine how to best tell that story. When working through the case and displaying images, it is essential to consider how the images appear to those watching your presentation:

- Choose studies which are most relevant to the current clinical question, with judicious use of comparison imaging
- Choose the window, phase or reconstruction that showcases the abnormality best e.g. using a coronal reconstruction to demonstrate the 'apple core' morphology of a primary colorectal cancer of the descending colon
- Manipulate the CT or X-ray window in real time if needed, e.g. adjust the soft tissue window towards a liver window on CT to better demonstrate liver lesions
- Scroll through stacks of images at a reasonable pace, pausing at the salient abnormality

If a presenter scrolls too quickly, the audience may be unable to follow as they are not expert radiologists themselves. If presenting online, the inherent lag of the connection may mean that following the verbal description is difficult.

Being questioned is part of the process and is not aimed to be argumentative or confrontational. Questions are often asked to seek important management information or demonstrate a clarify learning point. As MDT meetings are a valuable learning opportunity for all in the room, discussing interesting findings or imaging 'pearls' is a valuable exercise.

Should the imaging review meeting discover an error or discrepancy in a report, it should be fed back to the reporting radiologist. This conversation or communication is conducted with respect and humility, privately if possible. A written addendum should be added to the report to document the missed finding or report update (ideally authored by the original reporting/approving radiologist). The case can be recorded for upcoming discrepancy or mortality/morbidity meetings if appropriate.

BOX 2.6 PRACTICE QUESTIONS

- Define multidisciplinary healthcare and discuss the role of radiology within it.
- What is the role of the radiologist in a multidisciplinary team meeting?
- Outline the evidence for the effectiveness of the interstitial lung disease multidisciplinary team meeting and the potential impact on patient care.
- List three strategies to run an effective clinical meeting.

MEDICAL IMAGING LEADERSHIP SKILLS

Answering the question of 'what makes a good leader' is challenging, and there is no one correct answer or a summary of points that can be memorised. What we ask and require of our leaders is highly variable, with different traits and actions needed in different contexts and at different times. What's more, our cultural understanding of what good leaders look like is also constantly evolving, particularly as we strive to achieve greater diversity in our leadership bodies to better reflect the diversity of the population they serve.

Types of leadership

The business and medical literature presents many different models of types of leadership, noting the advantages and disadvantages of various styles in certain workplaces and specific situations. Individual leaders (particularly those who perform more effectively) may also change their leadership style to suit the changing nature of their work or move between styles as the circumstance demands. Different leadership styles are categorised by motivation and patterns of actions that leaders may exhibit. We will consider two models of leadership styles: one through the lens of emotional intelligence and the other a more practical behavioural classification of leadership.

Leadership styles and emotional intelligence

Daniel Goleman's model of leadership styles published in the *Harvard Business Review*[35] proposes six distinct leadership styles, which are linked to different facets of emotional intelligence:

- Coercive
- Authoritative
- Affiliative
- Democratic
- Pace-setting
- Coaching

When a leader uses a **coercive** style, they demand immediate compliance from their employees or fellow team members. A coercive style is generally considered one of the least effective leadership styles. Still, it can have a short-term role in crisis management and situations where decision action is needed. If a coercive leadership style is sustained, it can have significant detrimental effects on the culture of a department and individual team members, such as:

- Loss of a personal sense of value and pride
- Loss of a sense of initiative and motivation to engage and provide high-quality care
- Loss of faith in the goals/mission of the organisation
- Resentment of the leadership and/or organisation

An **authoritative** leadership style is one of the most impactful, focused on mobilising people towards a shared vision. The leader conveys a clear focus on the goal, why it is important, and how it relates back to the day-to-day work and contributions of individual team members. Underpinning this is a sense of why the work matters. Individuals are also offered greater flexibility; while the mission and shared goals are clear and fixed, how people achieve these aims is left up to them (within reason).

Affiliative leadership styles encourage the formation of emotional bonds and promote harmony between team members and the leadership. The philosophy is that people come first, expecting the time invested in building emotional bonds to be paid back in loyalty to the leadership and organisation. Ideally, the affiliative leadership style promotes idea sharing, freedom of work and a positive feedback culture. These approaches are beneficial in times when an organisation is forming or rebuilding.

However, using an affiliative leadership style in isolation can be detrimental to culture and performance. Poor individual or group performances may go uncorrected, and/or mediocrity could be inappropriately tolerated. A lack of a clear directive can also be detrimental to culture.

The **democratic** leadership style seeks to engage consensus in decision-making. Trust is built by investigating time and resources to collect individual ideas and engage in open discourse around the issues. Team members feel they have a stake in decision-making, and there is a greater propensity for setting realistic expectations. A democratic leadership style can be useful when a leader is uncertain about a decision or direction and requires fresh ideas and insights, but it is less useful in a crisis where decision and timely action are needed. The approach can be disadvantageous if over-consultation results in endless meetings and cycles of discussion. A meaningful democratic style also requires a team that is knowledgeable enough to provide relevant and informed contributions.

Pace-setting leaders expect excellence and self-direction from their team and exemplify these high standards. These leaders rapidly identify poor performers and issues and take decisive action. A pace-setting is often counterproductive, negatively impacting team culture and the team members who become disillusioned, disengaged and burnt out. Guidance is often unclear as the leader fails to articulate the standards required to the team members, and feedback is often minimal or of little value. Individuals can lose their sense of personal value and place within the team or organisation. "Micromanagers" fall into this category, where the leader is overly focused on details and steps in to perform the work of others too quickly if they deem it 'not up to standard'.

A pace-setting approach can work in some contexts in the short term, particularly if a specific project needs to be completed by a team of highly competent and motivated members. Even in this case, for pace-setting to be successful, it needs to be combined with other leadership styles.

Finally, the **coaching** leadership style aims to develop people for the future, helping team members identify their strengths and weaknesses and consider how they impact their current role and future practice. Through coaching styles, leaders take the time to provide feedback and more detailed instruction and engage in long-term goal setting. This style has perhaps the most significant positive impact on an organisation's culture and the individual team members; however, perception of the time and resources required to implement it present a barrier to its use.

As the approach focuses on personal development rather than results and outcomes, the benefits might not be visible immediately, even though they will become present with time. The coaching style requires continuous engagement and communication between leaders and team members, requiring an equal commitment from the individual to that of the leader.

These six leadership styles are best utilised in combination, with the flexibility to employ different styles at different times. This requires adaptability on behalf of the leader, with the emotional intelligence and insight to understand which style should be used and when to switch when a particular style is not working.

Leadership style models by behaviour

An alternative model of leadership outlines six distinct styles drawing from the behaviours exhibited by the leaders, adapted from the business world for the discipline of radiology by Narayan and colleagues.[36] These six leadership styles are:

- Transformative
- Transactional
- Authoritarian
- Laissez-faire
- Democratic
- Servant

A **transformative** leadership style contains elements of both the authoritative and coaching styles from the emotional intelligence-centric model, encompassing an inspirational style built on the foundation of a strong shared mission. Transformative leaders are often charismatic and utilise clear, open communication. This approach has been linked to higher levels of organisational productivity and greater creativity, innovation and engagement among team members. There are inherent risks of prioritising the team over the individual, who may not receive adequate guidance or be alienated in pursuing the higher goal. This style relies on a well-developed culture of mentorship and sponsorship for success.

Transactional leadership styles prioritise structure and clear definitions of roles and responsibilities. They also focus more on organisational rigidity, timelines, and the specific tasks required to reach the end goal or achieve the organisation's mission. This approach risks losing sight of the big picture and limiting the creativity and flexibility of individual team members. This, in turn, can negatively impact an organisation's culture, staff retention, individual performance, and, ultimately, community health outcomes.

When decision-making is performed exclusively (or near-exclusively) by a leader or leadership team, this is termed **authoritarian** leadership. This is not to be confused with authoritative leadership. In authoritarian approaches, no (or minimal) input is sourced from broader team members or the community served. This style risks enacting decisions that are out of touch with the culture and best interests of the broader team and the patient community. The approach is rigid and has been linked to creating a culture of mistrust and low morale.

The **laissez-faire** leadership style takes a more 'hands-off' approach to leadership, only intervening when the leader deems it necessary. This style is the most conducive to innovation, creativity, and flexibility. However, new staff may feel a lack of guidance at the outset, or there may be confusion among team members regarding the specific nature of their responsibilities. The laissez-faire style has been linked to high employee satisfaction and staff retention rates and improved motivation despite the relaxed atmosphere.

The **democratic** leadership style is essentially identical to that outlined in the emotional intelligence model. Through broader consultation and feedback processes, team members feel a stronger sense of shared ownership, trust and value. While the approach succeeds best at leveraging the skills and experience of team members, it relies on the team holding those skills and possessing sufficient experiential knowledge to make their contributions meaningful. Democratic processes risk losing time and resources through over-consultation and are less useful when urgent decisions are required.

Servant leadership styles are most strongly aligned with the principles of patient-centred care. This style prioritises the service of others above the leaders' personal interests. Leaders exercising this style invest in the professional development of staff in the interest of reaping long-term benefits for patients and the organisation more broadly. This style positively impacts culture, engagement, and value-driven care.

Inclusive leadership

Inclusive leadership styles ensure that employees feel their organisation values their perspectives and contributions. Inclusive leadership is considered a blend of other styles, building on the principles of diversity, equity and inclusion. It draws from the knowledge that workplaces that hold these tenants are often more efficient, culturally safe, and creative and deliver a higher quality of patient care. Inclusive leaders:[36]

- Value team members
- Invite diverse perspectives
- Recognise and support the contributions of a diverse range of employees

In practice, inclusive leaders should actively challenge ingrained processes and perceptions that promote 'sameness' across organisational practices and patient delivery. They challenge the status quo at individual, team, and organisational levels[36] and examine themselves for unconscious bias and challenging their own perceptions and beliefs.

The Diversity Council of Australia's model of inclusive leadership defines five inclusive leadership capabilities required for an individual to be an inclusive leader.[37] They need to be:

- Identity-aware (cognisant)
- Relational
- Open & curious
- Flexible & responsive
- Growth-focused

What makes a 'good' leader?

The perception of what makes a 'good' leader has evolved, echoing cultural change and the increased diversity of community and healthcare leaders. While favourable leadership qualities are traditionally skewed towards masculine attributes such as dominance, charisma, bravery and assertiveness, modern leadership analysis shows a greater appreciation of the more feminine communal traits. Communal traits include empathy, collaboration and transparency.

As there is variation in leadership style, there is also variation in the perception of what makes a good leader across teams, organisations and times. Favourable traits often include:[38]

- Authenticity
- Curiosity
- Analytical prowess
- Adaptability and flexibility
- Creativity
- Comfort with ambiguity
- Resilience
- Empathy

Leaders who fail to embody these qualities can have a range of negative impacts on the team and organisation. For example, if a leader is perceived as inauthentic, it can lead to mistrust among the team and degrade culture and relationships. If a leader is too rigid, it can stifle creativity, innovation, and curiosity.

It is a common misconception that individuals are born leaders. While some possess an innate drive or inclination towards leadership, leadership skills can be learned, developed, and refined. Even well-established leaders can benefit from ongoing education and refinement of their skills, which is particularly important given the changeable nature of radiology practice and healthcare in general. For example, today's leaders must demonstrate greater adaptability in the face of rapid technological change across medical imaging. They should not be rattled by uncertainties, such as how AI will become more entwined with practice.

With expanding educational programs and a greater understanding of the role of workplace culture in well-being, modern leaders need to exercise empathy with their team and be open to feedback. They should be curious rather than suspicious of differing perspectives and open to problem-solving in different ways.

BOX 2.7   PRACTICE QUESTIONS

- Discuss how different leadership styles may impact the culture of a medical imaging department.
- Outline the principles of inclusive leadership.

ROLE MODELS, MENTORS AND SPONSORS

As professionals in any industry, medical imaging doctors have people they admire, aspire to emulate or are inspired by. The culture of role modelling, mentorship and sponsorship is essential to the discipline's success, bringing in talented medical students and junior doctors, and helping them become successful radiologists.

Throughout my career so far, I have been privileged to have many role models, some wonderful mentors, and a few who have sponsored me as I work towards my professional goals. What is special about these aspirational relationships is that you are not trying to be identical to them. Even now, as a fully qualified radiologist and nuclear medicine specialist, I still have role models, informal mentors and a few people I would consider sponsors.

Professional practice offers the flexibility to take inspiration from different people and use their examples or advice to build a professional practice identity that is right for you. Radiologists have so much to gain by learning from others, but always keep in mind that these relationships are precious and can be fragile. It is important to exercise gratitude and respect, both as a mentor and a mentee.

Role models

A role model is someone you look up to and admire. You may want to emulate their behaviours, practices, or career trajectories – wholly or in part. Considering someone a role model is viewed as a marker of great respect, with role models typically being more established and experienced in their field.

Role modelling is a passive process on the part of the role models themselves, and there is no direct communication involved.[39] The aspirational figure may not know someone looks up to them and is working to emulate their behaviour.

There is no necessity for an established professional or personal relationship to exist in a direct form, but it can indeed exist. It is also common for doctors to have multiple role models based on different skills, behaviours or milestones. You may look up to one radiologist for how skilled they are with interventional radiology and another for their practical approach to neuroradiology. You may have role models outside of radiology practice, for example, a surgeon who is a wonderful educator or an organisational psychologist who urges you to reconsider your approach to work.

Role model relationships can evolve into mentor relationships.

Mentorship

A mentorship is established when there is active communication between a mentor and a mentee, with the goal of the mentor acting as both an advisor and role model to the mentee as they work towards their professional and/or personal goals.[40] These relationships require input from both the mentee and the mentor, as well as open communication over time.

Strong professional relationships benefit career development, with the mentor acting as a conduit for knowledge, resources, research and training opportunities. For junior doctors, radiology trainees, and junior consultants, a mentor can be especially useful in helping them navigate the complexities of training and professional practice. Mentors offer advice and inside knowledge across the broad scope of radiology practice, potentially exposing the mentee to new avenues to explore, training opportunities or different ways of thinking about a professional problem.

Mentor–mentee relationships can also bridge the gap between professional and personal, but only if sufficient trust has been built. Balancing professional and personal lives as a training radiologist can be especially difficult, given that the stressors of everyday work compete against knowledge acquisition, examination preparation, and home lives.

The potential advantages of having a mentor for the mentee include:[40,41]

- Improved skill and knowledge development
- Greater confidence and problem-solving skills
- Access to career opportunities
- Improved quality and volume of research output
- Increased likelihood of receiving research grants and funding
- Greater overall career satisfaction
- Reduction in stress and burnout

Benefits to the mentor also include reduced stress and burnout and greater job satisfaction. For the mentor, it is also personally fulfilling to guide and witness the eventual success of their mentee in achieving their goals.[41] Departments and organisations may experience higher staff retention rates and improvements in overall culture.[40]

Types of mentor relationships

Each radiologist's professional journey is unique; therefore, each mentoring relationship will be unique. Mentees may connect with numerous mentors at different times throughout their careers, each advising them about a different aspect of their professional or personal journey.

Mentorship relationships may be formal or informal. Formal mentoring programs are becoming more common in organisations and educational programs. For example, the consensus guidelines for programmatic assessment models in medical education specifically recommend that students have recurrent learning meetings with a mentor to discuss their learning journey.[42]

Formal mentorship programs are typically organised by a department, institution or organisation with the goal of improving culture or meeting specific organisational objectives. A mentor and mentee are paired together based on nomination or allocation. They are provided with specific objectives, and often a time period is specified.

A formal mentorship program in a radiology training program could pair a training radiologist with a consultant and recommend meeting once a month for a minimum of 30 minutes. For example, the objectives of this discussion would be the trainee's progress in their assessment requirements, preparation for exams, engagement with research and/or goals and aspirations for their career post-fellowship. The mentor can listen and offer advice based on their experiences. Short-term goals can be set to discuss at upcoming meetings, adding a layer of accountability to motivate the trainee.

A more junior doctor may proactively approach a senior staff member and ask them to enter a formal mentorship agreement, usually more structured with goals determined by the mentee. These relationships are typically established when the mentor and mentee have already made a personal connection.

Suppose the mentee chooses the mentor based on a personal or professional connection. In that case, it is advisable to work with and get to know them before embarking on a formal, longer-term mentoring relationship. This way, both the mentee and the mentor can decide whether the commitment is right for them.

Informal mentorships have little or no structure. They often grow organically from healthy professional or personal relationships as career advice and experiential knowledge are passed from the senior colleague to the junior doctor or student. The mentor and mentee may not even realise they have entered this relationship. Whether the mentorship relationship is formalised or informal, the same principles of gratitude and respect should be maintained.

Characteristics of a good mentor

Mentor–mentee relationships require the engagement of both parties. As such, the best relationships grow when the mentor is actively interested in helping the mentee grow professionally and personally. The mentee's success should be the relationship's shared purpose and goal.

A good mentor approaches communication openly and honestly, providing a psychologically safe space for the relationship to grow, be collaborative and accessible. The mentor should manage the expectations of the relationship, set boundaries and hold the mentee accountable where appropriate. A good mentor actively seeks feedback from the mentee regarding the process and whether it is working for them in moving towards their goals.[40]

What makes a 'good' mentor will vary based on the mentee. The ideal mentor is someone the mentee feels comfortable with, respects and admires. As mentorship is not about direct replication but fostering of growth, the mentor may be engaged for different reasons. They may possess a skill the mentee wishes to develop, have faced a similar challenge or have navigated a professional or personal path similar to what the mentee envisages for themselves.

Responsibilities of the mentee

While a two-way relationship is the hallmark of mentoring, the mentee should be responsible for initiating communication and arranging formal meetings. A proactive approach is best for success and also demonstrates to the mentor that their time and advice are valued.

At the outset, it is essential to remember that senior colleagues are not obligated to enter a mentoring relationship with you. This may be due to time, workload or resource constraints, discomfort with the mentoring process, or a perceived lack of chemistry. If they decline, this should be respected.

Formal mentoring relationships should only proceed should mutual agreement to participate be reached. Setting boundaries and expectations is useful at the start of the relationship; for example, it can help to agree on how frequently to meet, where the meeting should occur, and the scope of discussions. The mentee should be proactive in maintaining regular communication with the mentor and be mindful of the volume and frequency of communication.

When the mentor offers advice, the mentee should listen carefully and respect it. If the mentor suggests specific tasks, the mentee should act on these in a timely way and provide feedback at the next meeting. Should the mentee choose not to implement the advice, it is also important to discuss this with the mentor – explaining why the advice was not followed or the task was not completed. The feedback process is an important part of reinforcing the value of the mentor–mentee relationship, reassuring the mentor that the time and emotional energy they are investing into the mentee's success is worthwhile.

Structured mentorship meetings and goal-setting

The primary focus of the relationship is the mentee's professional and/or personal advancement. As such, it is best to embark on the mentorship partnership with a clear understanding of the mentee's goals and aspirations and how they envisage the mentor will help them attain them. Goals are not fixed and should be revised over time as the mentee develops and the relationship evolves.

The mentor and the mentee need to be clear about their expectations and limitations at the outset, and the mentor must be the primary driver of the sessions.

Formal mentorship meetings can be more efficient and effective if the mentee takes time to prepare. Preparation could include noting down a list of topics to discuss or specific questions to ask, or revisiting the short-term goals or tasks set by the mentor at the previous meeting. Any particular advice or suggested activities provided at the last meeting should be followed up at subsequent meetings. For example, suppose a mentor suggests the mentee get more information about a fellowship. In that case, the results of this search and reflections on the suitability should be discussed at the next meeting.

Challenges to successful mentorship

Numerous challenges to the success of mentorship relationships exist which can degrade the quality of the interactions.

The heart of the relationship is a mutual understanding of confidentiality and respect. If either the mentor or the mentee breaks this trust, it can cause significant damage.

The mentor's attitude towards the mentorship process is important in maintaining individual relationships and ensuring that they remain engaged with the mentorship of other junior staff in the future. Should they become disenchanted with the process, frustrated, or feel undervalued, they may choose to opt-out.

The commitment to mentorship also needs to be balanced against often busy professional and personal lives, particularly for the more senior staff members whose clinical time is financially valuable and in terms of workload management.

If a medical imaging department is not supportive of professional mentorship initiatives, it can represent a significant barrier to the success of relationships. This includes, in principle, support for mentorship generally and the practical provision of time and resources for mentorship discussions. Overall, mentorship relationships have a greater chance of a positive outcome should the organisation recognise their value.

Should a mentee engage more than one mentor, they must be wary of 'averaging mentors'. If more than one senior colleague is advising the junior on a specific professional goal, there is a risk that conflicting advice will cause confusion or indecision. Mentors may also become frustrated if they feel that the time they have invested is for naught if the mentee is also seeking the same guidance elsewhere.

Sponsorship

Sponsorship takes the mentorship relationship one step further. A sponsor not only acts as a mentor, but publicly advocates and seeks out opportunities for the junior mentee or protégé.[43] The aim is to not only provide advice to the protégé to help them reach their goals but also showcase them to the medical imaging community and increase their visibility. This will increase the chance of the protégé making meaningful academic or clinical connections and potentially expose them to opportunities and offers they may not have been privy to.

Benefits for the protégé include further increased job satisfaction, greater chance of promotion or recruitment for lucrative projects and higher confidence as they embark on professional practice or pursue professional opportunities.[43] As with mentorship, sponsorship relationships also have benefits beyond career advancement, especially the personal satisfaction of being part of the positive experience and sharing success.

Sponsorship helps departments and organisations discover, train and retain unrecognised talent. Effective sponsorship is linked to improved department culture, higher staff retention rates and improved quality of patient care and research outcomes. The professional connections forged in sponsorship can improve collaboration and respect across organisations.

Gender diversity and mentorship

Across healthcare and business sectors, men have traditionally had greater access to and success with sponsor–protégé relationships than women, with these discrepancies still persisting today. Given the professional and personal benefits of mentorship and sponsorship, this has often been flagged as one of the strategies to help address gender discrepancies in radiology workforces and subspecialty practice. Some challenges to the successful implementation of this strategy, often a combination of conscious and unconscious bias regarding women in radiology practice and leadership, and the expectations, pressures and constraints on women mentors.[44]

It is often desirable to pair women mentors with more junior women trainees based on shared experience and the mentee's ability to see aspirational qualities and common ground with their mentor. However, current workforce discrepancies and the demands of busy clinical workloads create a barrier. In addition, with fewer women mentors available or willing to participate in such relationships, there may not be enough mentors to go around without overburdening them with multiple mentees.[4]

Men can act as effective mentors to women; however, it is important to be cognisant of the challenges that may arise. The personal and professional challenges facing women in radiology are often distinct from those facing their male peers, particularly considering work–life integration, communication styles, and cultural/social expectations of behaviour. Men mentoring women must consider gendered differences when discussing career advancement strategies and providing advice.

If the male mentor approaches the relationship with a paternalistic motivation (often unconsciously), the mentor's biased perception of the capability or capacity of their mentee may impact the advice they give or opportunities they suggest. In addition, resentment or friction can result once the more junior woman mentee increasingly exerts professional independence or challenges the advice provided.[44]

The impact of intersectionality on women of diverse races and cultures must be considered within these professional relationships, as unique or magnified challenges are often encountered. Mentors must take time to consider the medical imaging profession and its inherent challenges from the perspective of the junior college. This way, more meaningful guidance and advice can be provided, and the strength of the relationship reinforced.

When mentor relationships break down

As valuable as mentoring relationships can be, they are not indefinite. As mentors and mentees grow and change, so does the relationship. If there is no longer enough value to be gained from the effort being put in, or if the interpersonal dynamic is no longer working, it is usually a sign to move on.

Suppose you, as a mentee, feel the relationship isn't working. In that case, the first step is to revisit the initial terms of the mentorship relationship, including the initial goals and expectations. Questions to ask yourself include:

- Have I achieved the goals I set for myself at the start of the mentorship?
- Have my goals changed, and, if so, is my current mentor still the right person to advise me?
- Is my mentor providing useful and effective advice to help me achieve these goals?
- Do I still feel comfortable engaging in open and honest discussions with my mentor?

If you have answered 'no' to one or more of these questions, it could be time to move on or re-evaluate the terms and expectations of the mentorship.

In cases where it is time to end the formal aspect of the relationship, it is best to do it in a timely way so as not to waste the time of your mentor or yourself. Things to keep in mind when approaching the end of the mentorship include:[45]

- Exercise gratitude and respect at all times
- Communicate the changing nature of your needs honestly rather than focusing on any perceived shortcomings of the mentor
- Be transparent and direct in discussion
- Leave things open so that things could be revisited in future – that is, try not to 'burn bridges'

The mentor may offer to re-adapt to your changing goals and needs or recommend a new mentor better suited to guiding the next stage of your career. It is worthwhile expressing to your outgoing mentor what you have learned and how they have helped you. If they leave the relationship feeling valued and respected, they are more likely to mentor others in future and/or continue to help you professionally should opportunities arise.

BOX 2.8   PRACTICE QUESTIONS

- 'Mentors and role models are important to the professional development of training radiologists.' Discuss this statement.
- What is the difference between a role model, a mentor and a sponsor?
- You have been in a formal mentorship with a senior colleague for 12 months. You are concerned that the mentor–mentee partnership is not helping you to achieve your professional goals. How would you approach this?

REFERENCES

1. Kenny L, Turner S, Johnson C, et al. *Radiating Change: A Vision for Diversity, Equity and Inclusion at RANZCR.* Royal Australian and New Zealand College of Radiologists (RANZCR): Sydney, 2023.

2. Lightfoote JB, Fielding JR, Deville C, et al. Improving diversity, inclusion, and representation in radiology and radiation oncology part 1: Why these matter. *Journal of the American College of Radiology* 2014; *11*: 673–680.
3. Diversity Council of Australia. The case for D&I, https://www.dca.org.au/resources/di-planning/business-case-for-di (2023, accessed 15 September 2024).
4. Ayesa SL, McEniery JC, Hill LS, et al. Navigating the glass labyrinth: Addressing gender diversity in Australian and New Zealand representative radiology leadership. *Journal of Medical Imaging and Radiation Oncology* 2023; *67*: 155–161.
5. Hayter CL, Ayesa SL. Female representation in radiology subspecialty interest groups in Australia and New Zealand. *Journal of Medical Imaging and Radiation Oncology* 2023; *67*: 162–169.
6. Wu X, Bajaj S, Khunte M, et al. Diversity in radiology: Current status and trends over the past decade. *Radiology* 2022; *305*: 640–647.
7. Malhotra A, Futela D, Khunte M, et al. Intersectionality and faculty compensation in academic radiology in US. *Academic Radiology* 2024: *31*(12)5228–5231
8. The Pride Network: The University of Sydney. Pride Network, https://www.sydney.edu.au/about-us/vision-and-values/diversity/pride-network.html (2024, accessed 26 September 2024).
9. Parra DA, Gladkikh M, Jones LM. Factors influencing teamwork in healthcare applicable to interventional and diagnostic radiology. *Clinical Radiology* 2023; *78*: 897–903.
10. Larson DB, Langlotz CP. The role of radiology in the diagnostic process: Information, communication, and teamwork. *American Journal of Roentgenology* 2017; *209*: 992–1000.
11. Katzenbach JR, Smith DK. The discipline of teams. In: *HBR's Ten Must Reads on Teams.* Boston, MA: Harvard Business Review Press, 2013, pp. 35–53.
12. Lee YD. Company culture is everyone's responsibility. *Harvard Business Review*, February 9, 2021.
13. Willis MH, Friedman EM, Donnelly LF. Optimizing performance by preventing disruptive behavior in radiology. *Radiographics* 2018; *38*: 1639–1650.
14. How to create a positive work culture in radiology. *Aunt Minnie*, https://www.auntminnie.com/industry-news/article/15631377/how-to-create-a-positive-work-culture-in-radiology (2022, accessed 24 September 2024).
15. Porter J. To improve your team, first work on yourself. *Harvard Business Review*, January 30, 2019.
16. McClintock AH, Fainstad T. Growth, engagement, and belonging in the clinical learning environment: The role of psychological safety and the work ahead. *Journal of General Internal Medicine* 2022; *37*: 2291–2296.
17. Deitte LA, Lewis PJ, Gadde JA, et al. Strategies to create a psychologically safe radiology learning space. *Journal of the American College of Radiology* 2023; *20*: 473–475.
18. Deitte LA, Lewis PJ, Gadde JA, et al. Strategies to create a psychologically safe radiology learning space. *Journal of the American College of Radiology* 2023; *20*: 473–475.
19. Billstein LE, Robbins JB, Awan OA. Teaching emotional intelligence: How much do we care about it? *Radiographics* 2021; *41*: E68–E70.
20. Arora S, Ashrafian H, Davis R, et al. Emotional intelligence in medicine: A systematic review through the context of the ACGME competencies. *Medical Education* 2010; *44*: 749–764.
21. Barnhill A. The 3 C's of building team loyalty. *Forbes*, March 23, 2023.
22. Erickson T. The biggest mistake you (probably) make with teams. *Harvard Business Review*, April 6, 2012.
23. Comcare. *Good Work Design: Building Trust in Your Team.* Canberra, 13 March 2024.
24. Porath C. No time to be nice at work. *New York Times*, June 19, 2015.
25. Almost J, Wolff AC, Stewart-Pyne A, et al. Managing and mitigating conflict in healthcare teams: An integrative review. *Journal of Advanced Nursing* 2016; *72*: 1490–1505.

26. Angelo E. Managing interpersonal conflict: Steps for success. *Nursing Management* 2019; *50*: 22–28.
27. Parikh JR, Harolds JA, Bluth EI. Workplace bullying in radiology and radiation oncology. *Journal of the American College of Radiology* 2017; *14*: 1089–1093.
28. Rawson JV, Thompson N, Sostre G, et al. The cost of disruptive and unprofessional behaviors in health care. *Academic Radiology* 2013; *20*: 1074–1076.
29. Murphy DR, Singh H, Berlin L. Communication breakdowns and diagnostic errors: A radiology perspective. *Diagnosis* 2014; *1*: 253–261.
30. Chinene B, Nkosi PB, Sibiya MN. Radiography managers' perspectives on the strategies to mitigate disruptive behaviours: A qualitative exploratory study. *Healthcare (Switzerland)*; *10*. Epub ahead of print 1 September 2022. DOI: 10.3390/healthcare10091742.
31. Gallo A. How to navigate conflict with a coworker. *Harvard Business Review*, September–October, 2022.
32. Jo HE, Glaspole IN, Levin KC, et al. Clinical impact of the interstitial lung disease multidisciplinary service. *Respirology* 2016; *21*: 1438–1444.
33. NSW Health. Multidisciplinary team - integrated care, https://www.health.nsw.gov.au/integratedcare/Pages/Multidisciplinary-team-care.aspx (accessed 18 August 2024).
34. European Society of Radiology (ESR). 'Role of radiology in a multidisciplinary approach to patient care': Summary of the ESR International Forum 2022. *Insights Imaging*; *14*. Epub ahead of print 1 December 2023. DOI: 10.1186/s13244-023-01377-x.
35. Goleman D. Leadership that gets results. In: Alan Hooper (Ed.), *Leadership perspectives*. Routledge, 2017, pp. 85–96.
36. Narayan AK, Boone N, Monga N, et al. Fostering organizational excellence through inclusive leadership: Practical guide for radiology leaders. *RadioGraphics* 2024; *44*: e230162.
37. Diversity Council of Australia. Inclusive leadership, https://www.dca.org.au/resources/diplanning/inclusive-leadership (2023, accessed 15 September 2024).
38. Knight R. 8 Essential qualities of successful leaders. *Harvard Business Review*, December 13, 2023.
39. Kostrubiak DE, Kwon M, Lee J, et al. Mentorship in radiology. *Current Problems in Diagnostic Radiology* 2017; *46*: 385–390.
40. Bredella MA, Fessell D, Thrall JH. Mentorship in academic radiology: Why it matters. *Insights into Imaging* 2019; *10*(1):107 DOI: 10.1186/s13244-019-0799-2.
41. Donovan A. Views of radiology program directors on the role of mentorship in the training of radiology residents. *American Journal of Roentgenology* 2010; *194*: 704–708.
42. Heeneman S, de Jong LH, Dawson LJ, et al. Ottawa 2020 consensus statement for programmatic assessment–1. Agreement on the principles. *Medical Teacher* 2021; *43*: 1139–1148.
43. Perry RE, Parikh JR. Sponsorship: A proven strategy for promoting career advancement and diversity in radiology. *Journal of the American College of Radiology* 2019; *16*: 1102–1107.
44. Bickel J. How men can excel as mentors of women. *Academic Medicine* 2014; *89*: 1100–1102.
45. O'Hara C. How to break up with your mentor. *Harvard Business Review*, May 29, 2014.

Responsible Practice

3

QUALITY IMPROVEMENT AND AUDIT

Patient harm in a healthcare setting is one of the leading causes of patient morbidity and mortality globally, with literature indicating that approximately half of patient harm is preventable.[1] The World Health Organization defines patient safety as:

> The reduction of risk of unnecessary harm associated with healthcare to an acceptable minimum... An acceptable minimum refers to the collective notions of given current knowledge, resources available and the context in which care was delivered weighed against the risk of non-treatment or other treatment.[2]

Patient, staff, and community safety are at the core of medical imaging practice. Detecting, acknowledging and managing diagnostic errors is essential due to clinical radiologists' central role in image interpretation. Other unique hazards that need to be accounted for in imaging departments include:

- Radiation safety
- Magnetic safety
- Administration of contrast agents
- Imaging-guided procedures

Errors and incidents

Broadly, an **error** in healthcare is when an action is not carried out as planned – occurring as a result of wrongdoing (commission) or neglecting to do the right thing (omission).[2] A **violation** is when there is a deliberate deviation from a planned action.

The Australian Clinical Excellence Commission defines a **patient safety incident** as any incident which is an unplanned or unintended event or circumstance which could have resulted, or did result, in harm to a patient.[3] Incidents can occur because an unplanned or unintended event happened during the care delivery, the outcome of an illness or management did not meet the patient's expectations, from a recognised risk

68   DOI: 10.1201/9781003466529-3

associated with a procedure or when the patient did not receive a treatment or intervention as planned.

Patient safety incidents can be classified as:[3]

- Harmful incidents (formally adverse events), where harm was caused to a patient as a result of the event
- 'No harm' incidents, where the event occurred, but no harm was caused to the patient
- Near-misses (or 'close calls'), where an error or potential hazard was identified and corrected before an event could occur

Patient safety incidents usually occur secondary to a combination of factors, including:[4]

- System and organisational factors
- Technological factors
- Human factors and behaviours
- Patient-related factors
- External factors

Errors resulting from human factors and behaviours are often a symptom of underlying issues at an organisational/system level or linked to other technological, patient or external factors. The most serious incidents are rarely the result of a single isolated error, more commonly attributed to multiple errors or system failures that occur together.[5]

In diagnostic radiology, harm can be caused if the error causes a delay in diagnosis, treatment initiation, or misdiagnosis. An estimated 3-5% of radiology study reports contain an error; however, the majority of these will not cause a clinically significant adverse outcome.[6] These errors can occur at different stages including:[5]

- Review, triage and protocolling of the imaging request
- Technical factors relating to the performance of the imaging study
- Missed or misperceived imaging findings
- Misinterpretation of imaging findings
- Delay in or failure to communicate critical findings to managing clinicians

Incident reporting

Incident reporting systems are now commonplace in healthcare settings worldwide and are mandated in public and private practice across Australia and New Zealand. The formal reporting, recording, and investigation of workplace near-misses, errors, and incidents are critical to ensuring that workplaces remain safe and that the highest quality of patient care is delivered.

An incident reporting system does not aim to be punitive. It aims to review the recorded events and consider how practices can be improved to minimise the recurrence risk. Reporting incidents also increases the staff's general awareness of safe working practices.

Most health jurisdictions will have their incident management policy, classifying recorded incidents according to their actual or potential severity and the risk of the event occurring again. Risk matrices guide managers in the action that needs to be taken in response.

The most extreme or severe reported incidents usually require a more thorough investigation and escalation to higher management and/or government levels. A Root Cause Analysis (RCA) is a structured method for investigating critical incidents. It aims to unearth the 'root cause' of the incident and propose recommendations to prevent further incidents and reduce the future risk of harm.

What is quality improvement?

Quality improvement (or quality assurance) activities and programs are designed and implemented to maintain and improve healthcare services and, ultimately, patient care.[7] Quality improvement is an ongoing process that includes reviewing clinical errors and incidents and the audit cycle. Importantly, it is not an exercise in blame or a review of an individual provider's practice.

From an organisational and system perspective, quality improvement initiatives exist to deliver the highest-quality care balanced against financial and resource considerations, ensure compliance with professional standards and meet accreditation requirements. From a professional perspective, clinicians also want to ensure that they are delivering the highest quality of patient care and are in line with current practice.[8] Quality improvement programs are required at all levels of clinical practice, although the nature of the program (including scope, involved staff and resourcing) will vary greatly.

Just culture

Just culture describes a professional environment where staff members feel comfortable discussing their errors and the errors of others, balanced against the recognition that high-quality patient care is the primary goal. Just culture does not discount the human factors in healthcare errors but considers them in a broader system context. Kruskal and colleagues write,

> A just culture recognises that even competent professionals make mistakes but does not tolerate disregard for risks to patients and misconduct. Such a culture should minimise fear among participants and should identify and introduce proactive, rather than reactive monitoring processes.[9]

The just culture model diverges from traditional error management cultures, focusing on human behaviour as the key factor. Just culture models move away from a 'blame' culture and encourage the identification of shortcomings within the system so they can be addressed collaboratively and fairly. It accepts that even the most competent practitioners can make errors and recognises that imperfect systems create error-prone environments. A just culture model requires:[8,10]

- Support from leaders both within the medical imaging department and the broader organisational structure
- Agreement with institutional governance policies
- Adequate training for supervisors and leaders regarding just culture principles
- Ongoing training and support for staff members, delivered consistently
- Regular time for review, discussion and improvement
- Involvement and support of all staff within the department
- Continued coaching and support of individuals and the team as a whole

The evidence for the success of the widespread implementation of just culture models in healthcare is mixed. In theory, the model hopes to increase error reporting rates and, through this, see an improvement in the quality of patient care as the causes of the errors are addressed. Although staff and departments broadly perceive a positive benefit, a review of error rates and patient safety outcomes in the United States questions whether there is a measurable value.[11]

Quality improvement and safety programs

Quality assurance initiatives can be classified as vertically or horizontally orientated, with both approaches required to build a comprehensive and effective quality improvement or safety program.[5]

Vertically orientated interventions target a specific issue implicated in a medical error – often one that has recurred or that has a higher risk of recurring. This may be a process or protocol, a technology or a piece of equipment or deficit in organisational or clinical knowledge. An example of a vertically orientated intervention would be an educational initiative focusing on education around hand hygiene before imaging-guided procedures to reduce post-procedure infection rates.

Horizontally orientated interventions aim to improve department culture more broadly. Initiatives targeted at improving culture aim to reduce the risk of human error, which could result in adverse events or patient harm. An example would be establishing a diagnostic reporting discrepancies meeting. A range of cases would be presented anonymously (without blame) for the purposes of peer review, feedback and education.

Quality improvement committees oversee the design, implementation and evaluation of safety and quality initiatives. The role of a quality improvement committee is to:[7]

- Assess and/or evaluate the quality of care, drawing on a range of data sources
- Identify problems or shortcomings in the delivery of care
- Make recommendations to address identified deficiencies
- Monitor the success of initiatives put in place to correct deficiencies

For a quality improvement program to succeed, it requires the following:[9]

- Institutional leadership and support
- A receptive departmental culture (just culture)
- Processes for managing patient and stakeholder relations

- A quality management team
- Continued engagement of all staff with the process
- Use of appropriate tools

Clinical audit

A clinical audit is a quality improvement activity encompassing a cycle of evaluating local practice, comparing this data with proven standards exemplifying high-quality care, and implementing strategies to improve local practice based on the findings. Effective audits do not exist in isolation but rather as part of a broader organisational program or culture of quality improvement initiatives with involvement from senior staff and healthcare leaders. Audit cycles are ideally repeated or ongoing to ensure the ongoing delivery of high-quality patient care.

There are four stages within each clinical audit cycle:[9,12]

- **Preparation and planning:** identifying and defining the process or problem, allocating/assigning staff members and resources, literature review and identification of existing standards, designing a protocol and selecting an appropriate method for data collection
- **Measurement of performance:** data collection, analysis of data, comparison of data against agreed standards, identification of areas of non-compliance with the audit standards
- **Implementation of change:** review of non-compliance to determine root causes, development of solutions/strategies to address, implementation of solutions/strategies
- **Sustaining improvement:** reanalyse data on patient outcomes after the intervention, repeating the cycle as necessary

All audit activities must be completed following local policies and procedures, respecting patient privacy, and maintaining ethical standards. Usually, clinical audits are registered with a local research office or other governance department. It is best practice to notify all staff and other stakeholders involved in the clinical service being audited in the preparation and planning phase.

The audit process begins with selecting a topic, which is usually based on the known or perceived needs of the service. Topics may be prompted by:

- An adverse event, 'no harm' event or near-miss
- Recognition of a clinical risk or patient safety concern
- Organisation or system needs (e.g. in anticipation of upcoming service chance)
- Complement staff professional development activities
- Recommendations from a regulatory body

Before authoring a research protocol, existing literature, guidelines, and relevant protocols should be reviewed.

Successful audit projects examine practices and processes that can be evaluated using robust data collection methods. They should hold the potential to recommend meaningful change if areas of non-compliance with audit standards are found.[12] The 'audit standard' is the 'gold standard' against which the local findings will be measured.

The audit standards will determine the patient population and the data collection type to be included in the audit. All details of the clinical audit should be recorded so that the steps can be replicated if the project is repeated.

Following data collection, audit results are shared with the clinical stakeholder group for review and discussion. Areas of non-compliance with audit standards need to be identified and discussed in this forum to unearth the underlying cause(s) for the non-compliance.

If underlying causes for non-compliance are identified, the audit team and clinical supervisors design strategies to address the shortcomings. Following approval by the group and local governance authorities, these initiatives are implemented under monitoring.

The final step of the audit cycle is re-evaluating the strategy/initiative, determining whether it has the desired positive impact on patient care, and formally documenting and sharing results. At this stage, governance and stakeholders consider whether the formal audit cycle needs to be repeated or continued.

Feedback and peer review

With the large volume of imaging studies reported daily, errors and discrepancies are an unfortunate but inevitable part of radiology practice. The focus becomes how to mini- mise the risk of clinically significant errors while committing to the continual educa- tion and upskilling of the radiology workforce. Peer review is one strategy to promote higher-quality service delivery and foster a continual learning environment for staff.

Peer review is an inherent component of radiology practice, often performed uncon- sciously by comparing previous imaging studies with the current examination or pre- senting cases at a multidisciplinary meeting or case conference.

Peer review is defined as 'the assessment of the accuracy of a radiology report issued by another radiologist',[13] and is not necessarily performed in a formal capacity. It also encompasses a review of interventional procedures, communication and the review of adverse events.[10] **Peer feedback** is how the peer-review findings are communicated to the original reporting radiologist.

Suppose a diagnostic imaging error or misdiagnosis has been found, particularly one with the potential to cause harm or change clinical management. In that case, it is best practice to communicate it back to the original reporting radiologist. If practical, any addendums to be made on written reports should come from the original reporting radiologist (it is not appropriate to addend the reports of others in most cases). Communication should be kind and considered, ideally undertaken privately if dis- cussed in person.

If a training radiologist or junior doctor has detected the error of a more senior radiologist, it is usually best to escalate the issue to a more senior radiologist (e.g.

clinical director, modality chief). This more senior staff member is better positioned to discuss the case with the original reporting doctor.

Finding out you have made a clinically significant error in your reporting can be a daunting and emotional experience for a radiologist. As such, these interactions should be handled with kindness, aim to uphold the principles of just culture and keep patient care as the primary focus.

Formal peer-review meetings and committees can be established to collect and review cases in the interest of improved service delivery and the education of members of the imaging department. These meetings ideally follow the principles of just culture, focusing on the context in which the error, event or misinterpretation occurred and potential contributors.[10]

BOX 3.1   FOR EXAMPLE …

An acute pulmonary embolism was not detected on a CT pulmonary angiogram study. When the imaging study is presented in a peer review meeting, the discussion could involve review of:

- *Technical limitations that may have impacted diagnostic accuracy e.g. timing of the contrast bolus/opacification of the pulmonary arterial tree, respiratory motion artefact*
- *Different imaging manifestations and appearances of common pathologies, complications and associated findings*
- *Associated imaging findings that may have obscured or distracted from the diagnosis, considering known sources of diagnostic error such as satisfaction of search*
- *Imaging interpretation techniques and approaches, e.g. search patterns, technical pearls*
- *The role any new technologies, protocols, software packages or AI could have in the case*

BOX 3.2   PRACTICE QUESTIONS

- You come across a fellow radiologist's report and notice an error that could impact patient management. How would you approach this?
- Briefly describe the clinical audit process as it pertains to clinical radiology.
- Outline the incident reporting system in your health service and describe its importance in maintaining quality practice.
- Outline the importance of the feedback process to maintaining the quality of clinical radiology practice.

MEDICAL IMAGING SERVICE DELIVERY, RESOURCE ALLOCATION AND FUNDING

Standards in imaging service delivery

Medical imaging service delivery is governed and held to account by standards of practice. In Australia and New Zealand, the standards of practice for clinical radiology are set by the Royal Australian and New Zealand College of Radiologists (RANZCR),[14] with further legislative requirements placed on practice by the governments of both countries. Standards of practice guidelines for nuclear medicine practice in Australia and New Zealand are outlined by several organisations, including RANZCR, the Australasian Association of Nuclear Medicine Specialists (AANMS) and the Australian and New Zealand Society of Nuclear Medicine (ANZSNM), again with oversight from the governments of both countries.[14-16]

Standards of practice govern all aspects of both diagnostic and interventional radiology service delivery, including personnel, facilities, equipment and practice management systems.[14]

Responsible practice initiatives and clinical decision-making tools

There is a widespread perceived issue with the overuse of imaging tests for unsuitable indications. The inappropriate use of diagnostic imaging tests can result in unnecessary risks to the patient from delayed diagnosis or radiation exposure, financial cost without benefit for the patient and the healthcare service provided and inefficient allocation of limited resources.[17]

For these reasons, medical imaging and broader healthcare organisations worldwide have created programs and awareness campaigns to assist referring clinicians and patients in more responsibly utilising imaging services (as well as other diagnostic tests and therapies). Typically, recommendations are created in the spirit of evidence-based medicine and evidence-based radiology, drawing from the consensus of expert clinicians and undergoing peer review.

Below are three such web-based initiatives. As radiologists themselves play a crucial role in educating our referrers about best imaging practice, it is worthwhile being familiar with the resources. I encourage you to visit the websites.

ACR Appropriateness Criteria®

The American College of Radiologists (ACR) Appropriateness Criteria® are evidence-based guidelines developed to assist referring clinicians in making the most appropriate imaging or treatment decisions for their patients' specific conditions.[18] The guidelines aim to improve the overall quality of patient care delivery and ensure the safe and efficient use of radiology services. The resource is web-based and undergoes peer review.

Recommendations consider specific clinical scenarios, assign an 'appropriateness category' based on the evidence-based and currently available technologies, and indicate the relative radiation level associated with the study in simplified terms. The Appropriateness Criteria categorise the study for the given scenario as:

- Usually appropriate
- May be appropriate
- Usually not appropriate

Despite the quality of the resources and the promotion on behalf of the ACR, there has been a reported low rate of incorporation of the guidelines into daily clinical practice.[19] This may reflect a lack of integration of the ACR Appropriateness Criteria® into formalised education programs for university-level medical students and training junior doctors, low levels of awareness among the referring clinician populations or perceived challenges with the website's user-friendliness.

www.acr.org/Clinical-Resources/ACR-Appropriateness-Criteria

Choosing Wisely

Choosing Wisely was an initiative of the American Board of Internal Medicine, which was developed to reduce the number of unnecessary tests, treatments and procedures for patients.[20] It focused on the education of managing clinicians so that they, and the patients they treated, would be better informed of the options available and were, therefore, in a better position to make decisions that minimised the risk of harm, maximised diagnostic utility, and did not incur unnecessary costs for the patient and/or health service. While radiologists and other imaging professionals can recognise when tests are being over-requested or utilised inappropriately, they cannot necessarily inform or influence the ordering habits of their referral base.[21]

Patient-centred care and informed consent principles were employed in promotional material, with patients encouraged to ask their treating doctors five questions:[20]

1. Do I really need this test or procedure?
2. What are the risks?
3. Are there simpler, safer options?
4. What happens if I don't do anything?
5. How much does it cost?

Radiology and nuclear medicine tests and procedures were a key focus of the campaign, with the American College of Radiologists one of the groups providing recommendations and feedback from the outset. In the early days of the campaign, there were concerns from radiologists that awareness of the campaign was not reaching a high enough proportion of referring clinicians and that the difficulties in accessing and utilising the lists of over-utilised studies.[22] The important role of radiologists in taking the initiative to educate their referring populations was highlighted as an important complementary measure, as was integrating the Choosing Wisely principles with the ACR Appropriateness Criteria®.

While the Choosing Wisely campaign in the United States has officially ended, multiple offshoot initiatives around the world have the same goal of reducing unnecessary tests and treatments. Choosing Wisely Australia, for example, promotes the goal of starting and continuing a 'national dialogue on unnecessary tests, treatments and procedures, and to support healthcare that is supported by evidence, not duplicative of other tests or procedures already received, free from harm (and) truly necessary'.[23]

www.choosingwisely.org
www.choosingwisely.org.au

Diagnostic Imaging Pathways

Originally developed by the Western Australian Government and now curated and hosted by Radiology Across Borders, Diagnostic Imaging Pathways (DIP) is 'an online suite of evidence-based and consensus-based imaging guidelines and an educational tool … to guide the appropriate choice of diagnostic imaging in clinical situations'.[17] Guidelines are presented as decision trees/flow diagrams for different clinical indications, considering the results of prior tests and clinical information.

DIP was initially rolled out across public health services in Western Australia, with additional dissemination of resources to selected general practitioners. Initial evaluations of the program in 2006 revealed that the pathways were found to be useful when clinicians were faced with unfamiliar scenarios or expert advice was not readily available.[24] Professional barriers were also noted, particularly in cases where senior medical staff would request imaging tests based on learned experience and gestalt. The initial technical access obstacles were overcome when the pathways were published publicly online.

www.radiologyacrossborders.org/diagnostic_imaging_pathways

Funding for medical imaging services in Australia

The cost of medical imaging service delivery in Australia varies depending on the practice setting i.e. whether the imaging service is part of a public health service or private enterprise.

Many medical imaging studies and procedures attract a government rebate when performed, regardless of whether the service is delivered in a public or private facility. These tests and procedures are typically well established in healthcare practice and have demonstrated proven benefits to patient outcomes. Some tests will only receive a government rebate if the patient is referred by a specialist clinician or if the referral is for a specific indication. For example, in Australia, there is a government rebate for patients undergoing FDG PET/CT for lung cancer staging. No funding is granted if the FDG PET/CT is referred for investigation of suspected infection.

Should a medical imaging test or procedure not attract a government rebate, the cost must be recovered elsewhere, e.g. through out-of-pocket payment by the patient, insurance coverage, or the hospital budget. If the patient is from overseas, the cost must be paid out-of-pocket or by insurance regardless of inpatient or outpatient status as there is no government provision. In private practice, the patient often pays an additional fee – even for scans that attract a government rebate. Individual practices set costs.

Whether funding is granted for a medical service or technology (including diagnostic imaging tests and imaging-guided procedures) is determined by the Medical Services Advisory Committee (MSAC).[25] Applications progress through preliminary screening and different committees to determine whether the service or technology should be publicly funded. The evaluation considers the safety, clinical efficacy and costs when making decisions.

The cost of medical imaging services can present a barrier to healthcare access for some groups and communities of patients. This is discussed in *Chapter 5: Cultural Safety, Advocacy & Emerging Technology.*

BOX 3.3   PRACTICE QUESTIONS

- Briefly describe the *Choosing Wisely* recommendations, including the aims of the initiative.
- Briefly outline how funding arrangements may impact a patient's imaging plan, using a specific example.

MEDICO-LEGAL ISSUES, QUALIFICATIONS AND CREDENTIALLING

Occupational health and safety

The fundamental principle that all workers have the right to a safe workplace underpins work health and safety. Guidelines, legislation, and policy regarding this will vary between practices, health districts, states and countries.

Occupational health and safety considerations in radiology encompass the risks associated with the healthcare environment and the unique risks associated with using different imaging modalities. Medical imaging departments will have their unique guidelines and policies to manage these risks but also work under the jurisdiction of broader healthcare and workplace safety policies. Risks and hazards that may be present in the medical imaging department include:[26]

- Radiation exposure, that is, for modalities that use ionising radiation such as X-ray, CT, fluoroscopy/angiography and nuclear medicine
- Magnetic risk (for MRI)
- Repetitive stress injuries, for example, shoulder injuries in sonographers
- Use of heavy lead aprons, such as those used in interventional radiology suites
- Ergonomics, for example, reporting workstation equipment and desk setup
- Body fluid exposure, including needle stick injuries
- Infectious patient exposure
- Manual handling (transport and moving of patients)
- Hazards of the physical environment, including slip and trip hazards

More than half of injuries to staff in the medical imaging department are sustained by radiographers, technologists and sonographers.[26] This is attributed to the physical requirements of the job and the requirement for frequent close patient contact. For sonographers, the physical act of scanning can increase the risk of repetitive stress injuries (e.g. to the shoulder) and infectious exposure.

The role of a **radiation safety officer** is to moderate radiation safety risk. They are responsible for ensuring staff compliance with radiation safety policies and practices and monitoring occupational radiation exposure.

Other strategies to assist in lowering workplace risk in a radiology department include:[26]

- Development of robust and clear safety policies
- Safety audits
- Walkarounds/visual inspections
- Safety reporting tools
- Employee education
- Fostering a culture of safety that promotes surveillance, reporting and management of hazards or potential hazards

Patient privacy and confidentiality

Patient privacy is the right of the patient to decide when and how their information is shared and to what extent others may access it.[27]

Confidentiality is upheld by those involved in providing care to the patient; that is, maintaining the patient's privacy by protecting their personal information. In medical imaging, this extends to protecting the right to privacy regarding medical images, reports, and documentation regarding diagnostic and interventional procedures. The patient has the right to have their information respected and protected.

Upholding patient privacy and confidentiality is important for the patient, their family, the organisation and the clinician. Privacy breaches can result in distress, embarrassment or damaging consequences. Breaches can lead to an erosion of trust in an organisation or medical imaging as a specialty and bring about reputational damage and legal action in severe cases. For the clinician responsible for the breach, disciplinary or legal action may result.

While privacy breaches can be deliberate, they also encompass less overt actions such as:

- Accessing medical files outside of the scope of work duties (including the records of oneself or family members)
- Discussing patient information within a public setting such as a café
- Inappropriately transferring patient data over personal email or data sharing systems

Patient privacy should be considered across data collection, storage, access, clinical, audit or research use and transfer. Where possible, patient identifiers should be removed.

Disclosure of information can only occur for the purpose for which it was collected or directly related to that purpose.[28]

The responsibility of radiology staff to protect patients from harm extends to upholding the privacy and confidentiality of information contained within radiological images and associated documentation.[29] As this information is stored online, the security of the patient's electronic medical record is vital in upholding confidentiality. The trade-off is that medical imaging professionals make quicker and more accurate clinical decisions when there is prompt and straightforward access to electronic patient records.

To uphold the high quality of patient care while maintaining patient confidentiality, radiologists and other medical imaging staff work within secure IT systems. It is the responsibility of the staff to ensure their training in the systems is up to date and that the training itself is robust and in line with local practice guidelines as well as broader privacy laws.[27]

Electronically stored patient information can be protected by:[27]

- Using data encryption
- Restricting physical access to authorised staff only
- Preserving copies and data backups
- Properly disposing of outdated devices and data storage
- Restricting off-site access through secure channels such as via virtual private networks (VPN)

Clear and accessible security policies should support these physical initiatives, with education and training for all staff.

Witnessing and identifying patient abuse and neglect

Radiology has a unique role in the detection and reporting of patient abuse and neglect. 'Red flag' indicators of abuse may be present on imaging only, with the radiologist's role to consider whether the imaging findings are concordant with the stated history or need further investigation. Patients of any age or gender can be victims of abuse, although radiology services play a particular role in the detection of physical abuse in paediatric patients. Diagnostic imaging may also play a role in the assessment of patients who are suspected victims of domestic violence or elder abuse.

As with all imaging reports, careful correlation with the patient history and clinical presentation should be performed during image interpretation. Should the reporting radiologist suspect that unreported physical abuse could be the cause of injuries detected on the scan, concerns should be discussed directly with the referring clinician. Conversations should be clearly and accurately documented in the imaging report, including with whom the conversation occurred and the time and date.

Outside of the reporting of medical images, doctors and healthcare providers, in general, are bound by mandatory reporting laws (noting the specifics of these laws will vary). Reporting should occur if there are reasonable grounds to suspect that a child is at risk of significant harm. These laws are in place to identify and escalate cases of suspected child abuse and neglect and have been created with the safety and welfare of the child as the highest priority. Confidentiality laws protect reporters of abuse, and they cannot be held legally liable for the notification they make.

Conflicts of interest

A conflict of interest is a 'situation in which a person is or appears to be at risk of acting in a biased way because of personal interests'.[30] In medicine, recognising potential conflicts of interest is critical, particularly if it threatens the delivery of optimal patient care.

The professional lives of doctors are not limited to the direct provision of patient care, with clinicians often developing relationships with organisations, institutions and financial companies across their careers. In some cases, financial relationships are born out of these professional connections – which is not necessarily a bad thing. A **conflict of interest** arises when a personal or financial relationship with one organisation could potentially impact the best interest of a patient, another organisation, or a research project.

Transparency and open disclosure about the relationship's nature can help manage a potential conflict of interest. If appropriate, a clinician may have to abstain from certain decisions, research or quality assurance projects, or practice activities should the conflict potentially impact impartial decision-making or care delivery.

Social media and clinical practice

Social media encompasses websites and online applications that allow users to create and share content and connect. Over the past decades, social media has become more integrated into medical and medical imaging practice to connect with colleagues, foster relationships, and access educational resources. Social media can also help boost a radiologist's public and professional profile and expand the opportunities for collaboration, research, and professional development. Online case-sharing sites such as Radiopaedia[31] allow dissemination and participation in educational resources and connect a broad community of medical professionals interested in radiology.

With the benefits of social media, there are potential pitfalls, including the dissemination of misinformation, inadvertent (or overt) public breach of patient confidentiality and the potential for conflict of interest to arise in the instance of financial gain.[32] Medical imaging professionals are inherently linked to their employing organisations and bound by their social media policies. Should an individual's posted opinions be at odds with an organisation's official values and guidelines, disciplinary action may result.

Social media gives healthcare consumers a public forum to post their views and concerns. Patients can publicly post their images and voice opinions on their medical imaging care, which can have implications for the organisation and the clinician if they are named.[33] Situations such as this are challenging as they pose professional and personal identity risks.

BOX 3.4   FOR EXAMPLE …

Should a radiologist find themselves in a situation where social media is used to highlight a perceived error or complaint against them, they should discuss the matter with their manager and be guided by local organisational policies and guidelines.

They should refrain from responding directly to the post via the social media platform.

Complaints on social media should be handled as any other complaint, with open communication and transparent escalation policies.

Radiologists as expert witnesses

An expert witness is a person who provides a report or gives evidence in legal proceedings (or otherwise) based on their specialised knowledge of the subject. The expert witness is not bound to provide only factual evidence. The evidence may be presented in the form of a written report and/or be presented in court. The role of the expert witness is to:[34]

- Examine and analyse the material provided
- Interpret the material provided to form an opinion based on their skills and expertise as a radiologist
- Communicate the formulated opinion to the legal counsel or statutory body that has commissioned the opinion
- Be available to provide an impartial opinion fairly and in the interests of justice

Radiologists who testify as expert witnesses are required to act objectively and ethically at all times. Opinions should not be presented as facts, and radiologists should avoid providing specialist counsel on areas outside the scope of their knowledge and practice. Confidentiality and privacy should always be maintained, and conflicts of interest should be declared transparently.

Registration and licensing

To practise as a specialist in clinical radiology and/or nuclear medicine, specific qualifications, registrations, and licences must be in place and current. Additional modality or study-specific qualifications may also need to be in place, e.g., certification for cardiac CT reporting.

In addition to possessing a medical degree from a recognised tertiary institution and fellowship with RANZCR, requirements to practise in Australia and New Zealand include current:[14]

- Medical registration with the national regulatory body
- License to supervise the operation of ionising radiation equipment
- Basic life support certification

Additional radiation licensing and training is required to be accredited to practise as a nuclear medicine specialist in Australia. In other jurisdictions, additional training outside the clinical radiology training program may not be required.

Continuing Medical Education (CME) and Continuing Professional Development (CPD)

Continuing Medical Education (CME) and Continuing Professional Development (CPD) are terms often used interchangeably to describe the ongoing education, training, and certification that radiologists need to pursue throughout their careers after completing formal specialty training. Some consider CME a component of CPD.

CPD is a requirement of practice to ensure that radiologists keep up to date with current knowledge and new technologies and imaging techniques in the interest of continually providing the best-quality patient care.[35] Beyond knowledge, CPD offers radiologists an opportunity to broaden their expertise, upskill in new areas and develop personal and professional skills. Medical professionals across all health disciplines must participate in CPD, or risk losing their medical registration/licence to practise.

The requirements for completion of CPD vary between countries and organisations. However, a set number of hours will require completion and guidelines as to what learning activities represent. For Australian and New Zealand radiologists, types of CPD activities include:[36]

- **Educational activities** e.g. research participation, attendance at conferences, courses or meetings, teaching or supervision
- **Reviewing performance and reflecting on practice** e.g. participating in peer review or professional governance
- **Measuring outcomes** e.g. participating in audit processes or clinical outcomes related to research

---

BOX 3.5   PRACTICE QUESTIONS

- Discuss the role of occupational health and safety in radiology, describing a clinical example.
- You would like to use a patient's image in a lecture. What steps would you take to maintain the patient's confidentiality?
- You identify several imaging 'red flags' for non-accidental imaging on a paediatric skeletal survey. Describe how you would manage this.
- Define a conflict of interest, giving one example.

- Briefly outline how a clinical radiologist may act as a defendant or consultant in matters of litigation.
- Describe the importance of Continuing Professional Development (CPD) to maintaining the quality of clinical radiology practice.
- Define and describe the levels of evidence as they relate to evidence-based practice.

MEDICAL IMAGING LEARNING AND TEACHING

Knowledge is built, maintained, and improved throughout a doctor's medical career to ensure the ongoing delivery of high-quality medical care to patients. This means that access to quality medical imaging educational resources and experienced educators is important throughout all professional stages.

To maintain safe and effective practice, radiology knowledge is essential not only for radiologists and radiology trainees but also for medical students and non-radiologist clinicians. Medical imaging will be part of most patients' journeys at some stage, whether at diagnosis, during the treatment and active management phase, or during the follow-up period. This means that most clinicians need to make decisions regularly regarding the utilisation of medical imaging investigations, the counselling of patients, and the explaining of results. In addition, most non-radiologist clinicians are required to interpret imaging studies at some stage during their clinical practice, either independently or pending review from a radiologist.

Radiology is a unique field, with knowledge constantly changing and updating. Being closely interwoven with technology and innovation, teachers must stay current with recent advancements and current practice standards to effectively provide evidence-based education. In the education space, there is the additional challenge of the rapidly evolving nature of content delivery. Over the past two to three decades, educational sessions have evolved from case presentations on static film to electronic presentation formats such as PowerPoint and via an online PACS (Picture Archiving and Communication System). Where lectures and tutorials used to be exclusively in-person, there are now growing options for decentralised learning through webinars, recorded lectures, virtual conferences and social media.

Medical imaging education

The unspoken agreement between the educator and the learner to collaborate and respect the process is at the heart of medical education. The learner needs to recognise the value of the experience and engage with respect and attention. The onus is on the teacher to deliver an experience that not only imparts clinical knowledge but also does so in such a way that the learner can process it and apply it to their current or eventual practice.

TABLE 3.1 Radiology education goals and principles for different learners

Medical students	Basic imaging skills: modalities, safety Basic interpretation skills Imaging in clinical decision-making Common and life-threatening diagnoses
Pre-vocational junior doctors	Revision and development of basic interpretation skills Imaging in clinical decision-making Practical imaging skills Common and life-threatening diagnoses
Training or specialist non-radiologist clinicians	Relevant modality interpretation skills Specialty-specific radiodiagnosis skills Analysis and evaluation of diagnostic imaging in a care pathway Diagnoses relevant to subspecialty practice
Radiology trainees	Progressive development of radiology medical expert and intrinsic/non-interpretive roles Higher-level interpretation and radiodiagnosis skills Understanding of imaging's role across all clinical settings Analysis and evaluation of diagnostic imaging in care pathways
Radiologists	Expert interpretation and subspecialty imaging skills/expert interpretation Continuing professional development

Broadly, medical imaging education can be divided into three main groups based on the target audience:

- Medical students
- Non-radiologist clinicians: pre-vocational junior doctors, training or specialist non-radiologist clinicians
- Radiologists: trainees/residents, qualified radiologists

Different learners have different requirements depending on their level of training, subspecialty expertise, and mode of engagement. As such, variable approaches and teaching methods will be required for various groups. The resources created and delivered for each group will differ in aim and scope, with some overlapping concepts and basic principles (Table 3.1).

Depending on the forum where the education session is delivered, the educator may need additional information technology skills, such as developing PowerPoint presentations, facilitating webinars, or utilising PACS systems for case presentations.

Who is teaching radiology?

Delivery of radiology education is variable across clinical and tertiary settings, with imaging skills often taught by a mixture of radiologists and non-radiologist clinicians. On the ward, learning is usually delivered by more senior colleagues within a learner's own specialty.[37] For example, a more senior respiratory physician or registrar teaching chest X-ray skills to an intern. Exposure to expert radiologists comes less frequently through requesting more complex imaging tests or multidisciplinary team meetings.

Even in some formal education settings, the commissioning of radiologists to teach medical imaging is variable. Barriers may include communication breakdowns leading to misconceptions regarding interest and engagement or a lack of connection between organisers and radiologist educators. Increasing radiologist workloads and rising rates of burnout have also hampered radiologist engagement in teaching.[38]

Radiologists and trainees should teach medical imaging to medical students and non-radiologist colleagues where possible, given that they are experts in their specialty. Taking ownership of education opportunities also allows radiologists to demonstrate their value as clinicians, break down stereotypes and misconceptions and present themselves as role models for those interested in the field. Further benefits of radiologists and training radiologists engaging in formal and informal educational activities include:

- Increased professional profile of medical imaging professionals in the healthcare community
- Greater visibility of radiology as a vocational option for medical students
- Greater respect and collaboration across subspecialties
- Development of grass-roots imaging skills at early career stages, which can be developed over time
- Improved patient flow regarding the appropriateness of tests and imaging-guided procedures
- Improved patient care through timely diagnosis and/or multidisciplinary decision-making
- Avoidance of perpetuating myths and misconceptions regarding imaging interpretation and radiology practice

The ability to teach is not a skill that is inherent in all medical graduates and must be cultivated and developed over time and with practice. As involvement in medical student and resident teaching is a requirement of specialty radiology training programs, it is imperative that radiology trainees engage in teaching opportunities.

Pre-vocational doctors and medical students interested in a radiology may also seek out teaching opportunities as a means of developing imaging skills and demonstrating an interest in the specialty. Care should be taken to ensure adequate supervision and mentorship by more senior radiology clinicians to ensure that accurate and relevant information is conveyed to learners. The mentor–mentee relationship in educational delivery has the added advantage of offering the more junior colleague the chance to learn imaging skills from the senior colleague and build meaningful professional connections.

Developing higher-level thinking skills

As clinician learners progress through medical school, then move into specialty training and post-fellowship practice, there is an expectation that they will progressively utilise higher-level skills in their education. The most common model to illustrate this is

TABLE 3.2   Bloom's *Taxonomy of Educational Objectives*.

Level 1: Knowledge (remember) *Recognising and retrieving facts from memory*	*What type of intravenous contrast is used for MRI studies?*
Level 2: Comprehension (understand) *Interpreting meaning from knowledge/facts*	*Explain the different contrast phases that could be used in a CT scan of the brain.*
Level 3: Application *Applying knowledge to new scenarios*	*A 35-year-old man presents with right iliac fossa pain and fever. Ultrasound demonstrates a distended blind ending tubular structure in the right iliac fossa which is tender to probe pressure. What is the most likely diagnosis?*
Level 4: Analysis *Break knowledge into its parts to make connections and draw conclusions*	*A 60-year-old woman undergoes MRI for characterisation of a cerebral lesion. Review the MRI sequences and determine the top three differential diagnoses. Justify your conclusions.*
Level 5: Synthesis (evaluate) *Critique and make judgements*	*Discuss the advantages and disadvantages of CT-guided percutaneous lung biopsy.*
Level 6: Creation & evaluation *Bring together knowledge to make something that is new and functional*	*Design an audit to review the diagnostic yield of lower limb Doppler ultrasound.*

Adapted from Smith et al.[39]

Bloom's *Taxonomy of Educational Objectives*, which structures a hierarchy of the types of thinking used to tackle learning tasks and develop higher-order skills.

Developing these higher-order application skills will allow the learner to successfully transition from medical school knowledge building to the complex clinical environment. While early medical school learners will focus on the lower levels (i.e. knowledge and comprehension), radiology trainees approaching fellowship exams will be expected to demonstrate a more significant proportion of higher-level thinking skills (i.e. synthesis and evaluation). Basic skills must be developed before higher-level skills to ensure that skills and knowledge are built progressively, and learners are not overwhelmed (Table 3.2).

Methods of educational delivery

Types of educational sessions and resources in radiology education include:[31,40]

- Live lectures (in-person, webinar or hybrid session)
- Recorded lectures and videos
- Case-read-out sessions (in-person, virtual or hybrid session)
- Interactive tutorials (active learning including flipped classroom sessions)
- eLearning modules and simulations
- Adaptive tutorials (personalised online tutorials)

- Interactive case playlists (e.g. Radiopaedia.org)
- Static reading materials (textbooks, case books, journal articles)

The rise of digital learning environments, accelerated by necessity during the pandemic, has irreversibly changed the traditional in-person style of radiology teaching. This has been supported by improvements in hospital and university digital infrastructure, with freely available and good-quality teleconferencing software for staff and students. With radiology already operating within a digital clinical environment, the discipline was well-positioned for this transition. The European Society of Radiology has recommended that e-learning radiology modules should be incorporated into all medical school curricula.[40]

The advantages of delivering lectures, tutorials and case review sessions in a virtual real-time format include:

- Bringing together learners across locations for centralised learning
- Increased accessibility for learners stationed in regional/remote sites
- Reduction/elimination of commute times for learners to attend sessions
- Flexible attendance for learners with scheduling conflicts
- Option to record webinar-style sessions for revision or distribution to absent learners
- 'Control screen' features allowing learners to directly interact with scrollable image stacks for case-read-out or other interactive sessions

Disadvantages can include the perception of disconnection between educator and learner and the lack of real-time feedback through verbal and non-verbal cues. The feeling of disconnection can be amplified by the physical and social distance of the webinar format, with learners at risk of feeling disengaged if they do not perceive the teacher's enthusiasm translated through the screen. There is also a greater burden on educators (or support staff) to promote an interactive environment. They may need to monitor chat boxes or consciously pause and invite participants to unmute microphones to ask questions. Technological challenges in delivering the presentation can also detract from the experience, such as educator IT literacy, software issues or network access/connectivity.

Characteristics of good educational resources

Medical students and clinicians are inherently busy, with competing demands on their professional and personal lives. This means that any education sessions and resources they engage with should ideally cover high-yield topics and be fit for purpose.

Information is considered **high-yield** if it represents a significant gain in knowledge or experience. What is considered high-yield will vary between learners based on their background knowledge and setting of practice. While a lecture on 'Approach to Interstitial Lung Disease' may be a high-yield experience for a pre-examination radiology trainee, it would be much less valuable for a medical student unable to assess a chest X-ray confidently or competently. Determining appropriate content requires understanding what the audience considers important (or should consider important).

A resource that is **fit for purpose** is designed in such a way that it satisfies the goals of the exercise. For example, consider a surgical resident attending an educational session to improve their basic chest X-ray interpretation skills. If the session is overpitched and only reviews difficult cases above their knowledge level, the surgical registrar will not get much out of it. Alternatively, if the session covered image interpretation skills, building to review pathology common in surgical patients or potentially life-threatening, they would find the session more valuable.

Formal learning resources should have clear learning objectives, with content built to match these. Outcomes should go beyond the simple imaging identification of pathology and consider integrating practical imaging skills, decision-making in different clinical scenarios, and cross-correlation of imaging with other topics such as anatomy and pathology.

For recorded lecture content, maintaining engagement can be challenging as the immediate direct connection between teacher and learner is lost. It is more difficult for the presenter to convey enthusiasm and interest through the recording; however, this is essential. Educators can improve the quality of engagement with these recorded lectures by:

- Ensuring adequate sound recording capability with good-quality audio and minimal background noise or distracting alarms
- Using a video or webcam stream (if available/appropriate)
- Varying vocal tone and pitch
- Using interactive elements to highlight pathology and important concepts e.g. animations, moving cursors/indicators
- Integrating scrollable cases in addition to static images (if available/appropriate)

Active learning and the flipped classroom

As of the mid-2020s, most learners across radiology training and university programs and early career radiologists will be within Generation Y (Millennials) and Generation Z, with birth dates ranging from the early 1980s to the early mid-2000s. These generations grew up intertwined with technology and have unique learning needs compared to their predecessors. This includes a preference for interactive learning opportunities and multimedia resources over the traditional didactic style of lectures, with a desire for increased flexibility and different perceptions of the feedback process. For Millennial learners especially, there is a general want of measured positive and negative feedback, with no feedback potentially perceived as negative feedback.[41]

The changing needs of the learners have seen a shift towards interactive sessions that engage **active learning** skills. In a classroom with an active learning approach, learners are engaged with tasks involving problem-solving, open discussion or case scenarios. Examples in a radiology learning environment could include live-case assessment and/or interpretation of case-based scenarios focusing on designing imaging plans for different patient scenarios. This learning style aims to involve learners in such a way as to promote the retention of key knowledge and skills, ultimately increasing the success of applying the content to a real-world clinical environment.

A **flipped classroom** approach is a type of active learning that employs a self-directed approach to learning basic facts, with the session used to reinforce the knowledge and employ higher-level thinking skills to maximise the educational value.[42] Students are provided with resources to review prior to the scheduled session, which may include recorded lectures or videos, eLearning modules or specific readings. Learners value the interactive and flexible approach to learning and ability to retain the resources for revision purposes.

The educator needs to ensure that preparation for the session is completed in advance to allow the timely provision of resources to the learners. The resources provided should add value to the session and be relevant to the specific learning goals. The steps required to design a flipped classroom session include:

1. Reflecting on whether a flipped classroom session is the best way to teach the material
2. Drafting the lesson aims/objectives and outlining the lesson structure
3. Finding or creating the resources for the students
4. Distributing the resources to the students well in advance of the session, with instructions on how to use them
5. Finalising the lesson plan, incorporating the basic knowledge/skills contained in the resources

Promoting a safe learning environment

A learning environment is made up of the physical (or virtual) space, the context in which the learning takes place, and the culture the learners and educators are a part of. The benefits of developing and maintaining a positive and collaborative learning environment include:[43]

- Increased learning efficacy
- Greater work and educational satisfaction
- Improved staff morale
- Reduced burnout
- Fostering a sense of personal fulfilment and value among educators

Despite the benefits in practice, maintaining a positive environment can be challenging. Staff educators need to sustain their interest and engagement with programs and be willing to commit to ongoing learning and innovative practices. This is increasingly challenging in a time where the escalating complexity of clinical radiology brings competing demands on a radiologist or trainee's time.[43]

Given the often-high-pressure learning environment of radiology training, maintaining the psychological safety of a learner is critical. As learning radiology requires a perpetual critical appraisal of one's skills and reflection on errors and misinterpretation, effective educational cultures must balance prioritising high-quality patient care with providing a safe space for learners to develop skills. Cultures that do not mitigate the feelings of embarrassment, shame, or fear amongst learners when they make mistakes are not considered safe and risk long-term detrimental effects on the mental health of learners and the provision of patient care.[44] This applies to both interactive formal tutorials and case-readout sessions, as well as informal learning and feedback provided at the workstation.

BOX 3.6   PRACTICE QUESTIONS

- Describe the importance of medical student imaging education to quality radiology practice.
- Outline the characteristics of a psychologically safe learning environment.

CLINICIAN WELL-BEING

This section discusses issues of well-being, wellness and burnout in a general sense. It is worth remembering that mental health disorders disproportionately affect doctors, though they have not been specifically discussed here. If you are struggling with your mental health, I urge you to seek assistance. In the first instance, speak to a trusted friend, family member or colleague and check in with your doctor. Many health services also have assistance programs to connect staff with mental health services. If you are experiencing a mental health emergency or crisis, please seek emergency medical assistance or reach out to a crisis support service.

If you are in Australia or New Zealand, Lifeline can be reached at the following numbers:

- Australia: 13 11 14
- New Zealand: 0800 543 354 (0800 LIFELINE) or free text 4357 (HELP)

What is well-being and wellness?

The World Health Organization defines well-being as 'a positive state experienced by individuals and society. Similar to health, it is a resource for daily life and is determined by social, economic and environmental conditions'.[45] Wellness is a similar, but not identical concept, defined as the practice of healthy habits to achieve good physical and mental health.

Well-being and wellness, and their association with clinician burnout, have been an escalating topic of conversation in radiology workplaces, training programs and the academic literature. Clinician wellness has been recognised as a contributor to the quality of patient care, with poor doctor well-being a threat to patient safety and healthcare organisations more broadly.[46] Given its potential impacts on individuals, organisations, and patients, it has grown as a pillar of health strategy and has been integrated into training programs.

Following COVID-19, the declines in self-reported radiologist and clinician well-being have increased. This is related to escalating pressures in stretched healthcare systems and the personal toll of the pandemic. The complexity of these issues means that they are not easily solved; however, proposed targets for intervention include:[47]

- Addressing reporting volume and workload excess
- Decreasing the proportion of inappropriate imaging studies
- Improving work–life integration (rather than work–life balance, which may be unattainable)
- Reducing administrative and paperwork burden
- Simplifying IT systems and processes
- Fostering interpersonal connections
- Encouraging and nurturing professional growth
- Working with leaders to develop inclusive and psychologically safe leadership styles

Burnout

Burnout is an extended state of mental, physical and/or emotional exhaustion and is not equal to 'overwork' but rather a product of unmanaged occupational and/or environmental stress. It is not formally classified as a medical condition but rather an occupational phenomenon that can manifest with symptoms such as:[46,48,49]

- Loss of enthusiasm for work
- Emotional and/or cognitive exhaustion
- Depersonalisation & disengagement
- Low sense of personal accomplishment and/or feelings of inadequacy

While burnout manifests across all industries, it is highly prevalent in healthcare – affecting over half of American physicians and over 60% of radiologists.[49] The number of medical imaging doctors affected by burnout appears to be increasing, especially after the COVID-19 pandemic. Burnout is experienced not only by qualified radiologists but also by trainees. Junior doctors may be more vulnerable to financial and emotional stressors, and have the additional added pressure of high-stakes assessments and career uncertainty. Burnout among doctors has been linked to increased medical error rates and decreased quality of patient care.

Burnout has become an endemic problem due to several factors, including increasing workloads and higher professional and personal expectations placed on us by ourselves and others.[50] The balance between work and life is more precarious, with financial stressors rising with the escalating cost-of-living expenses. Furthermore, should a radiologist feel that they are not adding value to their profession or the community or feeling underappreciated or prevented from achieving personal goals, burnout may be the result.[46] Specific challenges contributing to burnout in radiologists are outlined in Table 3.3.

TABLE 3.3 Factors which may contribute to burnout in radiologists.

Increasing workload	• Increasing numbers of studies to report • Increasing volume of images to review with each study • Self-editing requirements (typists replaced with voice recognition) • Competing responsibilities (reporting vs case review meetings vs educational commitments) • Inadequate staffing • Time targets for report turnaround time
Practice environment	• Shift in practice settings towards larger organisations and private companies • Suboptimal leadership styles and hierarchies • Escalating bureaucracy and paperwork requirements • Impedance to achieving professional goals (e.g. in research, education, administration) • Academic pressures (e.g. grants, publications) • Career stage, especially early career radiologists competing for positions
Communication & autonomy	• Poor intra- and interdisciplinary communication • Lack of appreciation and/or perceived lack of value • Lack of transparency in decision-making • Loss of professional autonomy • Perceived barriers to efficient and fair work practices
Work environment	• Physical isolation (e.g. single reporting rooms, remote reporting) • Transition to virtual communication rather than face-to-face • Reduction in direct communication with referring clinicians • Professional silos • Sedentary and stationary reporting practices • Reduced sunlight and natural environment interaction • Distractions from technology and colleagues

Adapted from Chetlen et al.[49]

Given the broad range of professional and personal factors that can contribute to burnout, the solutions are equally diverse. At an organisational or institutional level, any strategies aimed at improving departmental culture, promoting psychologically safe practices, and helping staff members feel valued will assist in reducing burnout rates among staff.

Recovery from burnout must also happen at a personal level, and a number of strategies can be tried individually or in concert. These are summarised in Figure 3.1. There are personal things that can be done to promote rest, relaxation, and reflection, but it is also advisable to check in with your local doctor and speak honestly with your personal support team.

If you are experiencing burnout or know someone who is, I encourage you to speak up and seek assistance. I recommend visiting theburnoutproject.com.au for practical advice and resources to start your journey to recovery.

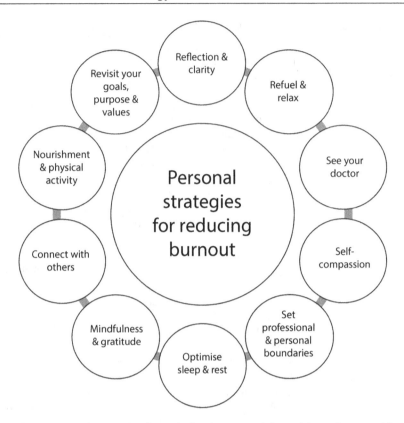

FIGURE 3.1 Personal strategies for reducing burnout. Adapted from *Burnout: Your First Ten Steps* by Dr Amy Imms.[50]

Work–life balance and work–life integration

Work–life balance and work–life integration can be used to describe the relationship between a doctor's competing professional and personal lives. The concept of work–life balance has been scrutinised recently, as achieving a 'balance' between clinical obligations and home life may be unattainable. The idea of work–life integration was thought to encapsulate better how the multiple facets of a doctor's life could be best woven together to promote well-being.

Either way, work–life balance and work–life integration are not static aims. The impact our professional commitments have on our personal lives (and vice versa) requires constant evaluation and adjustment.

Lupu and Ruiz-Castro[51] consider the pursuit of work–life balance as a cycle made up of five distinct steps:

1. Pause, reflect & reevaluate, e.g. ask, 'What is causing me stress, and how is this affecting my life at work and home?'
2. Pay attention to your emotions, e.g. ask, 'How am I feeling?'
3. Reprioritise, e.g. ask, 'What am I willing to sacrifice or change?' or 'Is this really necessary?'

4. Consider alternatives, e.g. ask, 'What are my priorities at work and home?'
5. Implement changes

Time management and getting things done

Developing time management skills is important for any training or qualified radiologist. Successful time management can increase the efficacy of reporting duties, integrate competing work tasks, and help with work–life integration. Jackson proposes that the five key steps to effective time management are[52]:

1. Set realistic goals
2. Get organised
3. Delegate tasks (where appropriate)
4. Relax and recharge
5. Stop feeling guilty

Two major barriers to the successful completion of tasks are procrastination and perfectionism.[52]

Procrastination is when a task (usually something daunting, distasteful or uninteresting) is delayed or postponed in favour of other, seemingly more attractive activities. The issue with procrastination is that if the less desirable task is put off, it can lead to escalating stress and anxiety, a greater workload in the days to come, and decreased quality of the final work. Overcoming procrastination is difficult, and successful strategies will vary between individuals. Some things to try include:

- Putting unpleasant and challenging tasks at the top of the 'to-do' list so they are tackled when the mind is fresh. Exciting or engaging tasks can be saved for later as a 'reward' for working on other tasks.
- Set realistic goals and small targets.
- Introducing accountability for completing less-desirable tasks by enlisting family, friends or coworkers or recording them electronically.
- Use timed-focus strategies such as the Pomodoro Technique. Plan a focused work session and set a timer (e.g. for 25 minutes). Remove distractions (such as phones), and work on the task with uninterrupted focus for the given time. Take a short (timed) break and repeat the process.
- Pick a study location that minimises distraction and maximises focus. For some people, this may mean a specific place in the home or the imaging department, or physically travelling to another location, such as a library or coffee shop.

Perfectionism is the refusal or reluctance to accept a standard of work that is anything less than perfect. The difficulty with perfection is that it is often not attainable, and those striving for it may use a great deal of time, resources, and emotional energy in its pursuit. This can drive anxiety and contribute to emotional strain and burnout. What's more, the task may never be completed.

A trade-off needs to happen between 'good enough' and 'perfect'; this balance depends on the circumstance.

For a diagnostic radiology report, identifying, describing and synthesising the clinically significant information is the primary goal – and, therefore, the standard of 'good enough' is quite high. In comparison, the stakes are less high for delivering a teaching session. Provided a good amount of effort is put in, these do not necessarily have to be perfectly prepared.

Interventional radiologists continually trade off 'perfect' for 'good enough', be that the position of the needle during a biopsy or the amount a vessel can be dilated with angioplasty. The decision to pursue 'perfect' has to be balanced against the risks to the patient of damaging a structure or prolonging an uncomfortable procedure.

Similarly, in life outside of work, we are allowed to give ourselves a break. The house does not have to be perfectly clean, and the lawn does not have to be perfectly mowed. Be kind to yourself.

To finish with my own mantra: 'Perfect is the enemy of done'.

BOX 3.7   PRACTICE QUESTIONS

- Briefly discuss the concept of clinician well-being, considering how it relates to radiology practice.
- 'Burnout' is an increasing concern in the radiologist workforce. Discuss this statement.
- Outline three strategies used to manage time effectively across professional practice.

REFERENCES

1. Panagioti M, Khan K, Keers RN, et al. Prevalence, severity, and nature of preventable patient harm across medical care settings: Systematic review and meta-analysis. *The BMJ* *366* (14185): 1–11.
2. World Health Organization: World Alliance for Safer Healthcare. *Conceptual Framework for the International Classification for Patient Safety*, http://www.who.int/patientsafety/taxonomy/ICPS_Statement_of_Purpose.pdf (2009).
3. Clinical Excellence Commission. What is a patient safety incident? In: *Open Disclosure Handbook*. Sydney: Clinical Excellent Commission, 2014, pp. 9–11.
4. World Health Organization. *Patient Safety: WHO Newsroom*, https://www.who.int/newsroom/fact-sheets/detail/patient-safety (2023, accessed 11 May 2024).
5. Donnelly LF, Dickerson JM, Goodfriend MA, et al. Improving patient safety in radiology. *American Journal of Roentgenology* 2010; *194*: 1183–1187.
6. Brady AP. Error and discrepancy in radiology: Inevitable or avoidable? *Insights Imaging* 2017; *8*: 171–182.
7. NSW Health. *Information Package for quality Assurance Committees Seeking Qualified Privilege - Under Health Administration Act 1982 Division 6b*, https://www.health.nsw.gov.au/factsheets/Pages/qualified-privledge.aspx (2018, accessed 11 May 2024).

3 • Responsible Practice   97

8. Broder JC, Cameron SF, Korn WT, et al. Creating a radiology quality and safety program: Principles and pitfalls. *Radiographics* 2018; *38*: 1786–1798.

9. Kruskal JB, Eisenberg R, Sosna J, et al. Quality initiatives quality improvement in radiology: Basic principles and tools required to achieve success. *Radiographics* 2011; *31*: 1499–1509.

10. Burns J, Miller T, Weiss JM, et al. Just culture: Practical implementation for radiologist peer review. *Journal of the American College of Radiology* 2019; *16*: 384–388.

11. Edwards MT. An assessment of the impact of just culture on quality and safety in US hospitals. *American Journal of Medical Quality* 2018; *33*: 502–508.

12. HQIP (Healthcare Quality Improvement Partnership). *Best Practice in Clinical Audit.* London, April 2020.

13. Strickland NH. Quality assurance in radiology: Peer review and peer feedback. *Clinical Radiology* 2015; *70*: 1158–1164.

14. Royal Australian and New Zealand College of Radiologists (RANZCR). *Standards of Practice for Clinical Radiology.* Sydney, https://www.ranzcr.com/college/document-library/ranzcr-standards-of-practice-for-diagnostic-and-interventional-radiology (23 July 2020, accessed 7 September 2024).

15. Australian and New Zealand Society of Nuclear Medicine. Quality and Technical Standards Committee Documents. *ANZSNM Website*, https://www.anzsnm.org.au/resources/quality-and-technical-standards-committee/ (2024, accessed 7 September 2024).

16. Australasian Association of Nuclear Medicine Specialists (AANMS). *AANMS Nuclear Medicine Standards.* Sydney, https://aanms.org.au/wp-content/uploads/2023/06/AANMS_NuclearMedicine_Standards_May2023_Final.pdf (May 2023, accessed 7 September 2024).

17. WA Government & Radiology Across Borders. *Diagnostic Imaging Pathways.* Radiology Across Borders, https://radiologyacrossborders.org/diagnostic_imaging_pathways/ (accessed 25 September 2024).

18. American College of Radiology. *ACR Appropriateness Criteria.* American College of Radiology, https://www.acr.org/Clinical-Resources/ACR-Appropriateness-Criteria (2024, accessed 25 September 2024).

19. Sheng AY, Castro A, Lewiss RE. Awareness, utilization, and education of the ACR appropriateness criteria: A review and future directions. *Journal of the American College of Radiology* 2016; *13*: 131–136.

20. ABIM Foundation. Choosing wisely. *Choosing Wisely*, https://www.choosingwisely.org/ (2023, accessed 25 September 2024).

21. Johnson PT, Mahesh M, Fishman EK. Image wisely and choosing wisely: Importance of adult body CT protocol design for patient safety, exam quality, and diagnostic efficacy. *Journal of the American College of Radiology* 2015; *12*: 1185–1190.

22. Levin DC, Rao VM. Reducing inappropriate use of diagnostic imaging through the choosing wisely initiative. *Journal of the American College of Radiology* 2017; *14*: 1245–1252.

23. NPS MedicineWise. Choosing Wisely Australia. *Australian Commission on Safety and Quality in Health Care*, https://www.choosingwisely.org.au/ (2024, accessed 25 September 2024).

24. Bairstow PJ, Mendelson R, Dhillon R, et al. Diagnostic imaging pathways: Development, dissemination, implementation, and evaluation. *International Journal for Quality in Health Care* 2006; *18*: 51–57.

25. Medical Services Advisory Committee. MSAC - MSAC Applications Process. Australian Government: Department of Health and Aged Care, http://www.msac.gov.au/internet/msac/publishing.nsf/Content/Factsheet-06 (2023, accessed 30 September 2024).

26. Siewert B, Brook OR, Mullins MM, et al. Practice policy and quality initiatives: Strategies for optimizing staff safety in a radiology department. *Radiographics* 2013; *33*: 245–261.

27. Radiological Society of North America (RSNA). Medical Information Privacy. *RadiologyInfo.org*, https://www.radiologyinfo.org/en/info/article-patient-privacy (2022, accessed 7 September 2024).

28. Information and Privacy Commission – New South Wales. Health Privacy Principles (HPPs) explained for members of the public. *IPC Website*, https://www.ipc.nsw.gov.au/health-privacy-principles-hpps-explained-members-public (2023, accessed 7 September 2024).

29. Andriole KP. Security of electronic medical information and patient privacy: What you need to know. *Journal of the American College of Radiology* 2014; *11*: 1212–1216.

30. Muth CC. Conflict of interest in medicine. *JAMA* 2017; *317*: 1812.

31. Gaillard F. Radiopaedia: Board of Editors. *Radiopaedia*, https://radiopaedia.org/editors (accessed 4 October 2022).

32. Júdice de Mattos Farina EM, Abdala N, Kitamura FC Social media platforms for radiologists: Perks and perils. *Radiology* 2023; *307*: e220974.

33. Ayesa SL, de Mattos Farina EMJ, Seidel RL, et al. The global reading room: Responding to a social media post. *American Journal of Roentgenology* 2024; *222*: e2329846.

34. The Royal Australian and New Zealand College of Radiologists (RANZCR). *Guidelines for RANZCR Fellows Who Act as Expert Witnesses.* Sydney, www.ranzcr.edu.au (November 2012).

35. Davis LP, Olkin A, Donaldson SS. Continuing medical education in radiology: A glimpse of the present and of what lies ahead. *Journal of the American College of Radiology* 2005; *2*: 338–343.

36. Royal Australian and New Zealand College of Radiologists (RANZCR). CPD overview. *RANZCR Website*, https://www.ranzcr.com/fellows/general/cpd-overview (2024, accessed 7 September 2024).

37. Butler KL, Chang Y, DeMoya M, et al. Needs assessment for a focused radiology curriculum in surgical residency: A multicenter study. *The American Journal of Surgery* 2016; *211*: 279–287.

38. Griffith B, Kadom N, Straus CM. Radiology education in the 21st century: Threats and opportunities. *Journal of the American College of Radiology* 2019; *16*: 1482–1487.

39. Smith EB, Gellatly M, Schwartz CJ, et al. Training radiology residents, bloom style. *Academic Radiology* 2021; *28*: 1626–1630.

40. European Society of Radiology (ESR). ESR statement on new approaches to undergraduate teaching in Radiology. *Insights Imaging* 2019; *10*: 109.

41. Chen P-H, Scanlon MH. Teaching radiology trainees from the perspective of a millennial. *Academic Radiology* 2018; *25*: 794–800.

42. The Derek Bok Centre for Teaching and Learning. Flipped classrooms. *Harvard University*, https://bokcenter.harvard.edu/flipped-classrooms (2023, accessed 25 September 2024).

43. Slanetz PJ, Reede D, Ruchman RB, et al. Strengthening the radiology learning environment. *Journal of the American College of Radiology* 2018; *15*: 1016–1018.

44. Deitte LA, Lewis PJ, Gadde JA, et al. Strategies to create a psychologically safe radiology learning space. *Journal of the American College of Radiology* 2023; *20*: 473–475.

45. World Health Organization. Promoting well-being. *WHO Website*, https://www.who.int/activities/promoting-well-being (2024, accessed 26 September 2024).

46. Fishman MDC, Mehta TS, Siewert B, et al. The road to wellness: Engagement strategies to help radiologists achieve joy at work. *Radiographics* 2018; *38*: 1651–1664.

47. American College of Radiology. *Doing More With Less: An ACR Well-being 360 Project*, 2023, https://www.acr.org/Member-Resources/Benefits/Well-Being

48. World Health Organization. Burn-out an 'occupational phenomenon': International Classification of Diseases. *WHO Website*, (2019, accessed 26 September 2024).

49. Chetlen AL, Chan TL, Ballard DH, et al. Addressing burnout In radiologists. *Academic Radiology* 2019; *26*: 526–533.

50. Imms A. *Burnout: Your First Ten Steps.* Hobart, Tasmania: AmyImms, 2019.

51. Lupu I, Ruiz-Castro M. Work-life balance is a cycle, not an achievement. *Harvard Business Review*, 2021, https://hbr.org/2021/01/work-life-balance-is-a-cycle-not-an-achievement (2021, accessed 30 September 2024).

52. Jackson VP. Time management: A realistic approach. *Journal of the American College of Radiology* 2009; 6: 434–436.

Research and Evidence-Based Radiology

4

ETHICS, INTEGRITY AND BIAS

Ethical research

Ethics in medical research is a broad topic that some academics dedicate years to studying. This section provides a brief outline of the guiding principles of medical ethics and expands on some important concepts.

Ethical research is much more than a checklist of what to do and what not to do. It encompasses acting with respect for those we work alongside and study, striving for outcomes that will contribute to the betterment of the world. What can be justified as being for the benefit of the population against the risk to the participant is often at the heart of ethical debate.

There are dedicated organisations in most countries responsible for producing local guidelines for ethical research practice. These comprehensive documents often form the basis for ethics applications and their review. In Australia, The National Health and Medical Research Council of Australia (NHMRC) is the governing body which produces the *National Statement on Ethical Conduct in Human Research*.[1] This document is regularly reviewed and updated. This body does not review research proposals specifically, with this falling to local Human Research Ethics Committees (HRECs).

The National Institutes of Health (NIH) defines seven guiding principles for ethical medical imaging research:[2]

1. **Social and clinical value:** the specific research question where the answer is important enough to justify the risk and/or inconvenience to the participants
2. **Scientific validity:** the specific research question is answerable and supported by sound research methodology
3. **Fair subject selection:** study participants should be recruited based on the scientific aims, not leveraging vulnerability or privilege

DOI: 10.1201/9781003466529-4

4. **Favourable risk–benefit ratio:** consideration of whether the hypothetical risk vs benefit of the study is acceptable and taking any possible steps to minimise risk
5. **Independent revision:** independent ethical review of the study proposal before it starts to minimise the risk of conflict of interest, bias and harm to patients
6. **Informed consent:** participants (both prospective and already enrolled) should be able to make their own decisions about whether to participate or continue to participate in the research based on the information provided
7. **Respect for potential and enrolled subjects:** participants should be treated with respect at all stages of the research study, whether or not they choose to participate, including the right to:

- Privacy
- Change of mind
- Being informed of changes to study protocols
- Welfare monitoring
- Feedback of study outcomes at the conclusion

The **informed consent** process is a key pillar of ethical research. The NHMRC[1] defines the 'requirement for consent' as participation in research is the result of a choice made by the participant. The requirement for consent has two conditions: that consent should be a voluntary choice and that this choice should be made based on sufficient information and understanding. The information provided to the participant should include the details of the proposed research and the implications of their participation in the study. Informed consent can be revoked at any time during the study. Some research studies can apply for a 'waiver of consent'; however, there are strict guidelines for this process.

Privacy (as it pertains to medical research) is the right of the participant to control access to their personal information and body. **Confidentiality** is a means of protecting the privacy of the participants, restricting the sharing and distribution of confidential, personal information. Inappropriate disclosure of information or use of data outside of the initial scope of consent is a breach of patient confidentiality.

Research integrity

Research integrity is the conduct of ethical research processes. It is underpinned by honesty, robustness, transparency and compliance with professional codes through all stages of the study, from proposal to reporting of findings.[3] Violations of research integrity include:

- Fraudulent research practices
- Reproducibility issues
- Questionable research methods and practices
- Inappropriate engagement with research enterprise

When research integrity is compromised, there is a risk of the broader community losing trust in the scientific community and misinformation spreading.

Bias in radiology research

Bias is a systematic error in the research process that can distort measurements and impact investigations. Ultimately, the results of the study can be impacted and the validity of the study degraded. The degree to which the validity is degraded is determined by the magnitude of the bias. Bias is present in all research, with some study designs more susceptible than others. Randomised controlled trials are considered the most powerful research methodology as they are the least vulnerable to the impact of bias through the strength of the randomisation process.

Systematic bias is different from random sampling error, which occurs when the sampling of the study population does not reflect the truth of the broader population. This is often the result of small sample sizes or study groups.

There are two broad categories of bias that are encountered in radiology research: selection bias and information bias.[4]

- **Selection bias** occurs when the characteristics of the study group are different from the characteristics of the broader population.
- **Information bias** results from differences in methods by which data is collected about or from the study participants.

Examples of selection bias in medical imaging research include:[4]

- **Sample bias:** when the target sample or control group does not reflect the characteristics of the target population
- **Loss-to-follow-up bias:** when the characteristics of the patients who do not complete the study to the specified endpoint differ from the characteristics of those who remain in the study
- **Disease spectrum bias:** when only cases within a limited spectrum of the disease manifestation (e.g. only patients with severe disease) are included
- **Referral bias:** when local practice preference impacts who is referred to and enrolled in a study
- **Participation bias:** when factors impact which patients reach the final stage of enrolment in the study
- **Image-based selection bias:** when the inclusion of a participants is subject to whether they have undergone a particular imaging study
- **Study examination bias:** when studies which are not considered technically adequate are excluded, resulting in the inclusion of subjects who are competent and well enough to undergo a technically adequate study

Examples of information bias in medical imaging research include:[4]

- **Interviewer bias:** when interview subjects are inadvertently 'coached' or led towards specific answers, or when medical records are only selectively reviewed
- **Verification bias:** when there are variations in how disease status is determined or when it is unethical to perform an invasive procedure to confirm a diagnosis in a patient where there is no suspicion of disease

- **Follow-up bias:** when participants with positive results undergo more intensive follow-up regimes than those who return negative results
- **Response bias:** variations in how accurately and thoroughly participants respond or non-random patterns of missing information
- **Reviewer bias:** a broad category of bias occurring when the person collecting information is not sufficiently blinded to the results of the reference test
- **Diagnostic-review bias:** when the reference test results are not definitive, and the results of the test under study play a role in the establishment of the final diagnosis
- **Test-review bias:** introduced in retrospective studies when the study test (or review of the test) has been performed after the diagnosis has been established; knowledge of the final diagnosis may impact interpretation
- **Incorporation bias:** when results of the test being studied are included as evidence for the final diagnosis
- **Read-order bias:** when studies are compared, and retained knowledge from a prior test impacts the interpretation of the next test
- **Measurement bias:** when there are discrepancies in measurement technique across studies, including variation in both subjective and objective measurements
- **Clustering bias:** when multiple measurements or observations of the index condition are made within a single participant
- **Context bias:** when the prevalence of the disease in the study population impacts measures of study accuracy
- **Publication bias:** where peer-reviewed journals are more likely to publish studies which return positive results or have high-quality study designs
- **Confounding:** when additional variables (known or unknown) impact the variable being tested

It is nearly impossible to eliminate bias completely in research studies. However, there are methods for reducing bias. These include **randomisation** of study groups (in prospective trials), preferencing **prospective** over retrospective study design and **blinding** of investigators.[4]

Blinding occurs when information is withheld from the investigators, e.g. patient outcome, demographics, and gender. In a double-blind randomised controlled trial, both the investigators and the subjects are blinded to whether they have been allocated to the intervention group or the trial group.

Plagiarism

Plagiarism compromises the quality of research and damages the credibility of the researcher(s) themselves and the scientific community more broadly.

Plagiarism is a form of academic misconduct, involving the appropriation of work that is not your own without acknowledgement. It is considered a serious academic offence in tertiary and literary circles, and disciplinary action can follow guided by the seriousness of the offence. Broadly, plagiarism is copying materials from another source without proper referencing or acknowledgement.[5] It includes copying written or spoken words, concepts or ideas, methodologies, images or artworks.

BOX 4.1   PRACTICE QUESTIONS

- Outline the guiding principles for conducting ethical research.
- Discuss the concept of bias as it relates to radiology research.

TYPES OF MEDICAL IMAGING RESEARCH

Qualitative and quantitative research

Qualitative and quantitative research both seek to understand and document the truth about the world around them. The difference lies in the differing philosophical definitions of that 'truth'.

The aim of qualitative research is to gain a greater understanding of the world in which we live, especially how people experience and behave in it and why. The qualitative researcher aims to consider meaning as it is shaped by individual context, experience and bias, illuminating the truth as the individual experiences it.[6] As such, truth is not absolute, and there can be multiple – equally correct – versions of it. The truth can mean different things to different people in different contexts and at different times. Qualitative research methodologies also accept that the investigators' inherent biases will influence the interpretation of the results. Qualitative research methods include:[7]

- Interviews and focus groups
- Observation of subjects
- Case studies of an individual, group of people or event
- Content analysis of written or multimedia material
- Narrative research, analysing personal accounts and stories
- Immersing oneself in the community being studied (ethnography)
- Active engagement with a community to bring about a change

In contrast, the quantitative paradigm assumes that the investigator and the subjects are independent and separate entities, unable to influence each other.[8] Quantitative methods are focused on numeric patterns, with data points measured or observed. The collected data undergoes statistical analysis. The goal is to analyse populations and determine causal relationships between variables, with the aim of reaching the most accurate representation of the one 'truth'. Participant sample sizes in quantitative research are often much larger than in qualitative research. Quantitative research is the dominant methodology in medical (including radiological) research.

Although qualitative and quantitative research methodologies seem to be two opposite sides of the coin, combining the two approaches to form 'mixed-methods' research protocols is common. In healthcare research, this approach is helpful as it provides a multifaceted analysis of the complex environment. For example, a study exploring the value of a medical imaging education program may incorporate quantitative data from pre- and post-assessments, as well as a thematic analysis of the attitudes of the participants based on short interviews.

Common research study designs

There are numerous different types of research study designs, which can be broadly divided into **descriptive** and **analytical studies**.[9]

The aim of **descriptive studies** is to gain a better understanding of what is happening within a given population, that is, to describe the nature of things. Descriptive studies include not only qualitative research studies but also case studies/series and quantitative survey studies, which document the characteristics of the population.

In contrast, **analytical studies** aim to quantify the relationship between two factors, comparing groups of patients that (ideally) differ by a single variable only. By doing this, the studies seek to determine whether an exposure, intervention, or treatment impacts outcome.

Analytical studies can be further divided into **experimental** and **observational studies**. In experimental studies, the investigator initiates the exposure, treatment or investigation, whereas in observational studies, the exposures, treatments or investigation will have already occurred, or will occur regardless of the study.

Randomised controlled trials are prospective experimental studies. Participants are allocated at random to receive a clinical intervention, often a treatment, to determine the effect of the intervention on health outcomes.[10] Participants are randomly allocated into study groups, ideally rendering the only difference between the populations the intervention itself. Randomised controlled trials are considered one of the most powerful study methodologies, with the strength of evidence produced from these trials being the randomisation process. Participant allocation is not influenced by the investigators or the patients, negating allocation bias.

Randomised controlled trials are not always ethically feasible or logistically possible. In these cases, observational studies are useful in evaluating the causal effect of a variable. Common study designs include cohort studies and case-control studies.

Cohort studies compare populations with and without a given exposure[11] – for example, studying the rate of post-angiography groin haematoma in patients who were managed with a vessel-closure device vs those who had manual pressure alone. Cohort studies can be conducted retrospectively or prospectively.

Retrospective cohort studies occur after all exposures, interventions and/or outcomes have occurred. In contrast, in **prospective cohort studies** the patients are identified at the time of exposure and/or intervention and are followed. Events are measured in chronological order to help distinguish cause and effect. Cohort studies aim to produce a 'risk ratio' which estimates the strength of the relationship between the exposure/intervention and the outcome.

Case-control studies select subjects based on their outcomes. The study groups are pre-existing, with one group consisting of patients who have had a given outcome, and a control group is taken from the broader patient population (often at random) who do not have the outcome. The exposure is assessed in both groups, aiming to quantify a causal link between the exposure and the outcome (i.e. does the exposure have a measurable impact on outcome?).[11]

BOX 4.2

TYPE OF STUDY	EXAMPLE RESEARCH PROJECT
Descriptive studies	
Qualitative study	An interview-based study on the attitudes and experiences of lung cancer patients engaging with medical imaging services.
Survey study	Reviewing the imaging studies and clinical data of patients who have lung cancer incidentally detected on CT pulmonary angiogram, and considering their demographics and clinical outcomes.
Analytical studies	
Experimental	
Randomised controlled trial	Randomly allocating patients undergoing biopsy to two groups, with one group receiving pre-procedural antibiotics and the other not. Infection and other complication rates between the groups will be compared.
Observational	
Cohort study	Comparing the clinical outcomes of patients on lung nodule surveillance who undergo FDG PET/CT scan in addition to CT, or CT alone.
Case-control study	Evaluating patients with newly diagnosed lung cancer, considering whether they were diagnosed through a screening program and the stage of the cancer at diagnosis. Is there a link between lung cancer screening and disease stage at diagnosis?

Systematic reviews and meta-analysis

Review articles are useful for collating results across multiple studies to pool knowledge and answer a specific clinical question. Systematic reviews were developed to bring a scientific approach to the review process, ideally minimising the bias and selective reporting encountered with traditional narrative reviews.[12] A **systematic review** aims to collate all the evidence for a specific research question, fitting within pre-defined eligibility criteria. The systematic methodology (as the name suggests) aims at reducing bias and giving rise to more reliable conclusions.

The Cochrane Collaboration is the most globally recognisable repository of systematic reviews and is the author of the *Handbook for Systematic Reviews of Interventions*.[13] They define that the key characteristics of a systemic review are:

- A clearly stated set of objectives with pre-defined eligibility criteria
- An explicit, reproducible methodology
- A systematic search that attempts to identify all studies that meet the eligibility criteria
- An assessment of the validity of the findings of the included studies, for example though the assessment of risk and bias
- As systematic presentation and synthesis of the characteristics and findings of the included studies

A **meta-analysis** extends the systematic review to combine the numerical results of all or some of the studies included in the systematic review. A meta-analysis produces an overall statistic summarising the impact of the intervention. This analysis may be performed to improve precision, to answer additional research questions, to create new hypotheses or to settle discrepancies across the literature.[13]

The PRISMA Statement was developed to assist the authors of systematic reviews and meta-analyses transparently report their justifications, methodologies and results.[14] The statement outlines a checklist of 27 items[15] which should be included in the review write-up to ensure systematic and sound appraisal processes are followed.

BOX 4.3   PRACTICE QUESTIONS

- Outline the difference between qualitative and quantitative research methodologies.
- Discuss the key principles, advantages and disadvantages of randomised controlled trials.
- Compare a systematic review and a meta-analysis.

CONDUCTING MEDICAL IMAGING RESEARCH

Research language and terminology

A basic understanding of the vernacular of research is required when reviewing, conducting, and even reading research studies.

A **hypothesis** is a statement about what you predict the results will reveal at the end of the study. It is not a research question, but rather what you believe the answer to the research question will be.

BOX 4.4   FOR EXAMPLE …

If the research question is "Does intravenous contrast improved the diagnostic accuracy of CT chest studies?", the hypothesis is "The accuracy of CT of the thorax is improved with the administration of intravenous contrast."

The **endpoint** is an important consideration in clinical trials. An endpoint is a targeted outcome that can be objectively measured to determine whether the intervention being studied directly benefits the patient. Examples of a clinical endpoint include disease-free survival, absence of disease, or resolution of pain.

The **outcome** of a research study is the results. Outcomes are variables that are studied and monitored during the research period, with the primary outcome that is most relevant to the research question being asked, and secondary outcomes additional variables considered to aid with the interpretation of the results. Outcome measures include:

- **Overall survival:** the length of time from diagnosis or commencement of treatment that the patient survives
- **Disease-free survival:** the length of time from diagnosis or commencement of treatment that the patient survives without evidence of signs or symptoms of their condition
- **Time to progression:** the length of time from diagnosis or commencement of treatment that the patient's disease grows or spreads to other parts of the body
- **Quality of life:** a complex concept which considers the overall well-being of the patient

Incidence and prevalence describe the rates of certain conditions within a given population. **Incidence** is the number of new cases during a specified time period. **Prevalence** is the proportion of patients living with the condition during a specified time period, regardless of when it was diagnosed.

When analysing the results of prospective randomised controlled trials, investigators often perform intention-to-treat and per protocol analyses.

The **intention-to-treat** analysis considers the results of all enrolled patients, regardless of whether they completed the study protocol correctly or not. Participants are assessed within the group that they were originally randomised into. Due to the impact of participant non-compliance, this analysis can underestimate the effect of the intervention being studied.

In comparison, **per protocol analysis** considers only subjects who completed the study protocol as written. This approach also risks introducing exclusion and other biases.

The **number needed to treat (NNT)** is the hypothetical number of patients who hypothetically need to undergo the intervention or treatment with one additional poor outcome, e.g., death or cardiac event. This gives an estimate of the treatment or intervention's impact on the patient population. The NNT must be balanced against the risk of adverse outcomes in clinical practice.

The hazard ratio, relative risk and attributable risk should be considered for therapeutic and interventional studies:

- The **hazard ratio** calculates how often an outcome occurs in one group compared to another.
- **Relative risk** is the probability ratio of an outcome occurring in the intervention group compared to the group that has not undergone the intervention.
- **Attributable risk** measures the proportion of the outcome occurring that can be attributed to the intervention.

Developing a research proposal

A proposal should outline the justification for conducting the research (the why) and the research question, how you plan to answer it, and the expected outcomes (the what). Research proposals will vary in style, length and composition depending on the institution you are preparing the proposal for; however generally require information on the research questions, methodologies, resources required, timeline and feasibility. The guidance below has been adopted from the University of Sydney,[16] summarised in Figure 4.1.

The **front matter** of a research proposal includes the project title, details of the team members, and supervisor/s. Some projects will require details of the proposed mode of the research.

The **aims and objectives** section will outline the scope of what you are trying to achieve through the project e.g. investigating a gap in the literature, conducting further study into an existing area of research, seeking to validate or disprove theory. The stated aim should be focused, clear and realistic statement. The objectives break down the aim into the steps needed to reach the intended outcome. These should be presented in a logical order.

This is followed by a concise **synopsis** outlining what the research is about, and a more expansive **background** section. The synopsis should explain in clear language the key aspects of why the study is being performed, how it will be performed and what the outcomes are expected to be. The background section provides context to the project, referencing a brief review of the current literature. The background should mention key research studies and contributors to the area of proposed study.

A section on the **expected research contribution** will describe why the research is being conducted in greater detail. It will consider the gaps in the current literature or justify why certain topics warrant further exploration. The investigator needs to communicate why the research question is worth asking, what the contribution to practice could potentially be, and demonstrate that it is innovative and original.

The section on the proposed **methodology** for conducting the research concisely explains the techniques that will be employed during the study, including the materials

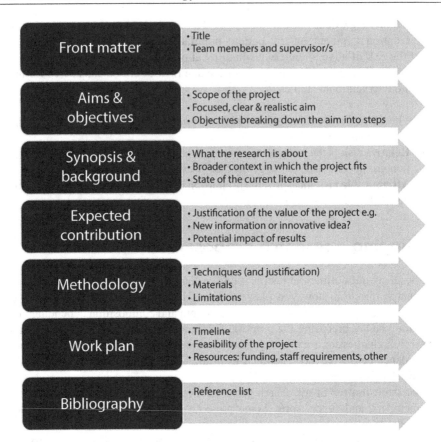

FIGURE 4.1   Parts of the research proposal. Adapted from The University of Sydney.[16]

and resources required. The choice of methods must be justified as appropriate to answer the research question, and any potential limitations must also be considered. Writing a methods section is covered in greater depth in the next section.

The outline of the **work plan** is crucial to the proposal, giving an overview of the timelines and feasibility of the research. It is of particular importance where timelines for completion are limited, for example, for research projects that need to be completed in radiology training programs or research degrees. A list of the **resources** required to carry out the work plan should be included in the proposal, detailing the nature of potential financial, staffing, or material resources needed to conduct the research.

Finally, a referenced **bibliography** of the citations mentioned throughout the proposal is required. This can be included at the end of the document or within the relevant section e.g. background.

Once a research proposal has been authored, it should be reviewed by the academic supervisor and other members of the team with relevant changes made prior to submission.

Reporting research findings

Research findings can be reported in several ways, including conference or scientific meeting proceedings (e.g. presentations or posters) or publication in peer-reviewed journals. Where a study's findings are reported will vary depending on the nature of the research question, scale and scope of the research, and strength of the research.

A research manuscript is typically broken down into seven sections:

- Title page
- Abstract
- Introduction
- Methods
- Results
- Discussion
- References

The **title page** contains the project title, as well as a list of the contributing authors and their academic and/or clinical affiliations. The corresponding author should be identified with contact details included. A title page often includes statements regarding potential conflicts of interest and ethical declarations.

The **abstract** is a summary of the study, usually structured as per the remainder of the report (i.e. introduction/aims, methods, results, conclusion). It generally does not contain references. The abstract should concisely outline the key features of the study and, ideally, should be understandable as a standalone. If the research is being entered into a conference, an abstract is usually submitted for review and may be published as part of the conference proceedings if accepted.

The **introduction** contains information about why the research is being conducted, as well as the project's aims and objectives. It often includes a brief review of the current literature, written to provide context for the research study and background knowledge. The gaps in the research and other justifications for conducting the study should also be included in the introduction.

The **methods** section details how the study was conducted and is crucial for judging the validity of the work. This section is particularly important in medical imaging research, given that scientific studies often involve technical imaging protocols. Information to include in the methods section include:[17]

- Details of regulatory approvals, including ethics approvals, registry details (for clinical trials and prospective studies), financial support and the consent process
- Details of the use of artificial intelligence (AI) technologies in the preparation of the manuscript
- Study design and participants
- Definitions of terms (if applicable)
- Imaging protocols used, described in sufficient technical detail to allow replication

- Details of the reference standard and index test (for diagnostic accuracy studies)
- Details of how images or results are read or analysed, including the number of readers and how they were blinded, and the software used in the analysis
- Summary of the statistical analysis, including the types of tests and analyses and details of any subgroup analysis

The description of the study design and participants should include the *who, where, when and what* of the research.[17]

The *who* is the population that was studied. The methods section should outline the sampling methods employed to recruit participants or how patients were selected for inclusion in the case of retrospective studies. The inclusion and exclusion criteria should be clearly outlined.

The *where* is the setting for the research, e.g. a single centre or across multiple centres. Depending on the manuscript submission process, the specific institution's name may need to be redacted for blind review.

The start and end dates of the data collection +/- patient recruitment constitute the *when*.

The *what* is the data that was analysed. Aspects of the study which need to be detailed include:

- Primary and secondary outcome measures
- Variables analysed, including interventions, exposures or comparative tests
- Whether subgroup analyses were pre-planned or post hoc (for RCTs only)

The **results** section reports the information gathered and analysed during the study, the output from the research methods. The results should directly answer the research aims outlined in the introduction.

In the **discussion** section of the paper, the author explores the meaning and relevance of the results as they relate to the population being studied, existing literature and the specific research question. In this section, evaluation and synthesis should be evident, with findings contextualised. New data obtained through the study should not be included in the discussion.

A short conclusion can be included to summarise the outcomes and their relevance to the broader community. The paper is concluded with a **reference** section, with in-text citations expected through the body text. Referencing should follow a recognised academic style (e.g. Vancouver, Chicago, APA) and be consistent throughout.

Submission for peer review

Once the research manuscript has been authored, it may be submitted to a journal for peer review. Selecting the journal for submission should be done in collaboration with the research supervisor to ensure an appropriate avenue for submission. Each journal will have its own set of guidelines for the preparation of a manuscript, which need to be followed stringently.

Following the submission of a manuscript through an online portal, the editorial board will consider the paper and determine whether it will progress to peer review. This decision is usually based on the quality of the research and manuscript, suitability for the journal (e.g. based on readership and content), and originality of the work.

The peer-review process ensures that published research maintains a high standard of quality, validity and originality. Reviewers are independent assessors and work under the guidance of the editorial board. Reviewers will make suggestions and recommendations, which editors review to make a final decision. The outcome of the review process is communicated to the manuscript authors, which may be acceptance, rejection of the paper or resubmission following major or minor revisions.

BOX 4.5   PRACTICE QUESTIONS

- List three outcome measures used in radiological research.
- You wish to study the complication rate for patients undergoing ultrasound-guided liver biopsy at your institution. How would you design this study?
- Describe how you would create a research proposal for a radiology study.

RESEARCH STATISTICS IN BRIEF

Statistical analysis in research is a broad and complex topic, far beyond the scope of a short guide. This overview of statistical principles and terms is not comprehensive. It aims to give an overview of the key terms and concepts necessary for evidence-based radiology practice and provide the basic tools to understand the clinical evaluation of diagnostic tests.

Definitions and terms[18]

Measurements of central tendency within statistics are the mean, median and mode:

- **Mean:** the average of values in the dataset
- **Median:** the middle number in the dataset when the numbers are arranged in order
- **Mode:** the most common value in the dataset

The **range** of a dataset defines the difference between the highest and lowest values.

A **normal distribution** (also known as a Bell Curve or Gaussian distribution) is a graphical display of data that resembles a bell. The graph is highest in the centre and then tapers outwards. The mean, median, and mode are theoretically the same value in a normal distribution.

Variables are the parameters measured in a study. They include characteristics, numbers or quantities that can be counted or measured. **Data** is information about the variables.

Descriptive statistics describe the data, presented as either numerical or categorical data. Descriptive statistics give information about the study population alone, and do not compare or correlate variables. **Numerical data** (as the name suggests) is presented in number form, whereas **categorical data** is a collection of data which is divided into two or more groups.

Numeric variables can be divided into continuous and discrete variables. In **continuous variables**, observations and measurements can take any value within the study range – down to the smallest increment that can be measured. Tumour volume is an example of a continuous variable. A **discrete value** is a whole number which cannot be fractionated. For example, a discrete value would be the number of pulmonary nodules detected on a scan (as you cannot have half a nodule!).

Categorical variables can be divided into ordinal and nominal variables. **Ordinal variables** can be divided into categories that can be logically ordered. An injury/severity grading scale or staging classification system would be an example of an ordinal variable. In contrast, nominal variables can be classified into categories, but those categories cannot be organised into a sequence, e.g. histological tumour types.

Probability is used to quantify uncertainty in research outcomes. It is defined as the relative frequency of an outcome occurring over a (hypothetical) infinite number of trials. The probability of an event occurring ranges from 0.0 (it cannot occur) to 1.0 (it will certainly occur). *P*-values and confidence intervals are measures of probability.

Inferential statistics are used to test how generalisable study results are to a broader population. They assist the researcher in drawing conclusions from their results and making predictions about their applicability to the broader population.

The **null hypothesis** states that there is no statistically significant difference between two groups of variables and that any observed difference is within the range of statistical variation. Most research studies aim to disprove the null hypothesis.

The concept of the null hypothesis is key to understanding hypothesis testing and the role of some common statistical tests. Investigators can use statistical tests (below) to calculate a P-**value** (*P* representing probability) to determine whether the observed difference in outcomes between the two groups is real or due to chance. If *P* is less than 0.05, the null hypothesis is rejected and the difference between the groups is interpreted as real. However, a difference does not automatically indicate causation.

A **type I error** (or false positive) occurs when a researcher rejects the null hypothesis, despite it being true within the population. A **type II error** (or false negative) occurs when a researcher does not reject the null hypothesis despite it not being true in the population.

Power is analogous to sensitivity and is the probability that the null hypothesis will be rejected when it is, in fact, false. The study's power is related to sample size, and complex calculations are available to determine the minimum sample size required (**sample size or power calculations**). These calculations consider the impact of type I & II errors, the effect size (see below), and expected variation within the sampled population.

Effect size represents the strength and magnitude of a relationship between variables, giving information as to how meaningful the observed difference between groups is. The effect size **confidence interval** allows generalisation of the study results to a broader population. The 95% confidence interval expresses that should the study be repeated, there is a 95% chance that the outcome would be the same.

Common statistical tests and their applications[18]

Statistical tests are employed to compare numerical data sets to determine the relationship between variables, calculating P-values and confidence intervals.

t **tests** compare the means from two groups, requiring numerical data, which has been sampled randomly and conforms to a normal distribution (i.e. Bell Curve). A paired *t* test is most commonly used to compare average differences of outcome variables in a single sample after an intervention. In contrast, a two-sample *t* test is used to compare the mean differences between two different groups.

A **one-way ANOVA** is similar to a *t* test in that it compares means between groups. It is used when there are more than two groups that require comparison. *t* tests and one-way ANOVA can be used to generate a P-value to help determine the statistical significance of the difference between the groups.

Correlation between groups can be tested with the **Pearson correlation test**, which seeks to evaluate whether a linear relationship exists between two groups of continuous variables. The results of Pearson correlation tests are expressed as the Pearson correlation coefficient (r). The r value will be between -1 and $+1$. -1 indicates a perfect inverse correlation, and $+1$ indicates a perfect direct correlation. When r is 0, it indicates the absence of a relationship between the variables. Note that Pearson correlation tests can only be used for the evaluation of linear relationships and can be unreliable if there is a non-linear component to the relationship.

Categorical variables can be analysed with **proportion analysis tests**, such as the Chi-square test, the Fisher exact test and the McNemar test. The **Chi-square test (X^2 test)** tests the frequency distribution of categorical data to determine whether the outcome is different from expected. It is useful for the analysis of large datasets. The **Fisher exact test** determines whether the distribution of data observed in two or more categorical variables is random. It is useful for smaller sample sizes. The **McNemar test** is used to compare paired variables, for example, comparing two imaging tests that have been performed on the same subject.

Assessing the accuracy of diagnostic studies

Sensitivity and specificity are the key measures of the inherent accuracy of a diagnostic investigation, and one should not be reported without the other.[19] **Sensitivity** is the probability of a positive result if the patient has the target condition, and **specificity** is the probability of a negative result if the patient does not have the target condition.

BOX 4.6   FOR EXAMPLE ...

Let's consider the accuracy of ultrasound in the diagnosis of acute appendicitis. The *sensitivity* is the probability that a patient with acute appendicitis will be correctly diagnosed on ultrasound.

The test's *specificity* is the probability that a patient without appendicitis will return a negative ultrasound study.

Sensitivity and specificity are considered alongside true and false positives, and true and false negatives. The relationship is shown in Table 4.1.

- **True positives** occur when patients with the condition are correctly classified
- **True negatives** occur when patients without the condition are correctly classified
- **False positives** occur when a scan is interpreted as positive when the patient does not have the condition
- **False negatives** occur when a patient with the condition returns a negative test result

Sensitivity and specificity can be calculated by considering these values:

$$\text{Sensitivity} = TP / (TP + FN)$$

i.e. positive tests in patients with the condition divided by the total number of patients with the condition;

$$\text{Specificity} = TN / (TN + FP)$$

i.e. negative tests in patients without the condition divided by the total number of patients without the condition.

This table also calculates the positive predictive value and negative predictive value. The **positive predictive value (PPV)** is the likelihood that a positive test reflects a

---

TABLE 4.1   True and false positives, and true and false negatives

		CONDITION	
		HAS THE CONDITION	DOES NOT HAVE THE CONDITION
Test result	Positive	True positive (TP)	False positive (FP)
	Negative	False negative (FN)	True negative (TN)

positive diagnosis, while the **negative predictive value (NPV)** is the likelihood that a negative test reflects a negative diagnosis.

$$PPV = TP / (TP + FP)$$

i.e. positive tests in patients with the condition divided by the total number of positive tests;

$$NPV = TN / (TN + FN)$$

i.e. negative tests in patients without the condition divided by the total number of negative tests.

Where sensitivity considers how likely the test is to detect the condition in a patient with the disease, positive predictive value considers how likely a positive test indicates the disease.

BOX 4.7   FOR EXAMPLE ...

A patient undergoes an FDG PET/CT for staging of lung cancer.

The *sensitivity* of the study considers how well the PET/CT detects involved lymph nodes.

The *positive predictive value* considers how likely an avid (hot) node on PET/CT indicates the presence of disease spread.

Accuracy is calculated by combining sensitivity and specificity into a single index measurement.[18] The number of true test results (that is true positives plus true negatives) is divided by the total number of tests:

$$Accuracy = (TP + TN) / (TP + TN + FP + FN)$$

This calculation of accuracy considers that there is a single threshold at which a positive diagnosis can be made.[18] In real practice, there may be multiple decision thresholds or a spectrum of imaging findings that represent the condition being studied.

Having a single threshold for positive diagnosis also does not consider the impact of disease severity on the investigation's results. More severe conditions usually have more pronounced imaging findings and are, therefore, more likely to be detected on the imaging test. Early or mild cases may have subtle imaging findings only, which may be more difficult to detect. Relying purely on sensitivity and specificity measures can over-simplify and introduce errors.

Receiver-operating characteristic (ROC) curves address this, incorporating a range of sensitivity and specificity data without a specific 'positivity threshold'.[20] Conversely, every possible decision threshold is considered with sensitivity and false positive rate (1 – specificity) data plotted against each other to give a visual representation of the data. This allows a review of the trade-off between these variables at different thresholds. This is considered the only valid way of comparing two diagnostic imaging tests.

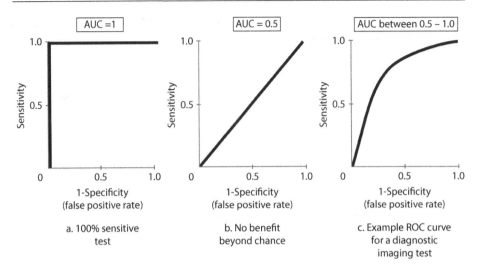

FIGURE 4.2   Examples of ROC curves.

The y-axis contains sensitivity, and the x-axis the false positive rate (1 – specificity). A perfect test would be correct in all cases (100% sensitive) with no false positives. A curve for such a diagnostic test is shown in Figure 4.2a. If a diagnostic test yields no benefit beyond chance (you could flip a coin with the same diagnostic accuracy), then the ROC curve would be a perfect diagonal (Figure 4.2b). In reality, a diagnostic test may not have perfect accuracy and may return a curve such as in Figure 4.2c. This curve can be used to find the optimal trade-off point between sensitivity and specificity.

The **area under the ROC curve (AUC)** allows investigators to compare different diagnostic tests. It is a broadly applied measure of the accuracy of diagnostic investigations. The closer the AUC is to 1.0 (a perfect test), the greater the accuracy of the test. The closer the AUC is to 0.5, the less discriminating ability it holds.

BOX 4.8   PRACTICE QUESTIONS

- What is the difference between the sensitivity of a study and its positive predictive value?
- Define a receiver operator curve and describe how it might be utilised in radiology research.

PRINCIPLES OF EVIDENCE-BASED MEDICINE AND EVIDENCE-BASED RADIOLOGY

Evidence-based medicine (EBM) is where clinical decision-making is based on the integration of current best evidence with clinical expertise and patient values.[21,22] EBM was introduced as a paradigm in the early 1990s by the McMaster Medical School (Canada) and has been adopted globally as a principle of best practice across all disciplines of medicine. It considers that clinical reasoning should be based, foremost, on valid, high-quality, ethical research rather than the anecdotal experience of individual clinicians. An EBM approach aims to ensure that decisions are made based on the highest quality knowledge, optimising the quality of care provided.

By extension, evidence-based radiology (EBR) provides diagnostic and procedural imaging services based on current best evidence, considering the patients' values and the local expertise and context. EBR encompasses the broader principles of EBM but also considers imaging-specific challenges related to patient safety and the operation of a busy department across a diverse range of modalities.

The implementation of EBM is achieved through 'top-down' and 'bottom-up' approaches, with the bottom-up approach more applicable to the local practice of radiology departments and the work of individual clinicians.[21] In top-down EBM, experts in high-level institutions review the evidence, formulating guidelines or 'white papers' to guide practice on a large population scale. In contrast, bottom-up approaches to EBM/EBR integrate high-level research with local clinical expertise and patient values, achieving standards better suited to local imaging practice and expectations.

Levels of evidence

A hierarchical system of classifying evidence from the literature is important to the practice of EBM (Table 4.2).[23] The hierarchy considers the strength and validity of certain study methodologies and their overall value weighting in the context of practice. A study with a stronger methodology, such as an RCT, is higher in the hierarchy than studies with less robust methodologies whose results are more susceptible to the impact of bias. This concept is linked to but distinct from the Pyramid of Evidence in evidence-based practice, which will be covered in the next section.

TABLE 4.2   Levels of evidence of therapeutic studies.

LEVEL	TYPE OF EVIDENCE
1a	Systematic review of randomised controlled trials (RCTs) with homogeneity
1b	Single RCT with a narrow confidence interval
1c	All-or-none study
2a	Systematic review of cohort studies with homogeneity
2b	Individual cohort studies or low-quality RCT
2c	Outcomes-based research
3a	Systematic review of case-control studies with homogeneity
3b	Individual case-control study
4	Case series or low-quality cohort study
5	Expert opinion without explicit critical appraisal

Adapted from Burns et al.[23]

Evidence-based practice model

The McMaster University model of evidence-based practice (EBP) involves five steps:[21,22,24]

1. **Ask:** formulating a focused and answerable question based on the clinical problem
2. **Search:** conducting a literature search, considering the hierarchy of evidence
3. **Appraise:** critically evaluating the selected evidence for validity, strength and clinical relevance
4. **Apply:** contextualising the results within clinical practice
5. **Evaluate:** reviewing and reflecting on the EBP process in regard to its extent, effectiveness and applicability to practice

Radiology trainees and residents may be asked to incorporate this approach into their formal training through a *Critically Appraised Task (CAT)*.

Step 1: Ask

When completing step 1, formulating a clear clinical question can be aided by using the PICO format:

- **P (Patient/Population):** who are the people whose care will be impacted by the review?
- **I (Intervention):** what test or intervention is planned for the patient?
- **C (Comparison):** what are the alternative tests or interventions, and what is the current standard?
- **O (Outcomes):** what would you like to achieve through the intervention or test? E.g. improved diagnostic accuracy, shorter recovery time, lowered complication rate

The question should be clearly defined and realistic for the investigator's skill level, scope, and resource availability.

Step 2: Search

A thorough search of the literature follows the initial question formulation, with the success guided by the clarity and applicability of the question. Searches will employ databases and other reservoirs of current evidence, and while there is a clear methodology to the search it is not as rigid or in-depth as prescribed in a systematic review or meta-analysis. The search for the best evidence ideally follows three steps:[24]

1. Identify search terms to fit the question
2. Search for secondary sources
3. Search for primary sources

The classification of 'primary' and 'secondary sources' is determined by the *Pyramid of Evidence*. Originally comprising 4 levels, the pyramid has grown over subsequent revisions to become the '6S Hierachy'.[25] Moving from top to bottom of the pyramid evidence is classified as:

- **Systems** e.g. decision support systems
- **Summaries** e.g. evidence-based clinical practice guidelines and textbooks
- **Synopses of syntheses** e.g. evidence collections such as Radiopaedia.org
- **Syntheses** e.g. systematic reviews
- **Synopses of studies** e.g. evidence-based abstraction journals
- **Studies** i.e. original articles published in peer-reviewed journals

The hierarchy of evidence will be applicable in different ways across EBR. For example, systems evidence at the top of the pyramid is best as a quick reference for real-time clinical decision-making. In short, the closer the evidence is to the top of the pyramid, the greater the ability to guide clinical management.[26] Higher levels of the pyramid integrate EBM from lower levels to progressively synthesise and summarise the evidence surrounding a specific research question.

Primary sources are the base of the *Pyramid of Evidence*, found by searching databases such as PubMed, EMBASE, and Google Scholar.[24] The quality of these primary sources is variable, and the investigator is responsible for appraising the evidence to determine its reliability and validity.

Secondary sources are the upper layers of the *Pyramid of Evidence*, the result of other authors scoping, appraising and collating relevant literature to provide a more cohesive answer to a research question. In the broader medical community, resources such as the *Cochrane Library* exist to collate review articles on a wide range of topics. Higher up the pyramid, online radiology resources serve the imaging community more specifically.

Step 3: Appraise

In the appraisal step, the selected article is evaluated for its validity, strength of evidence, and relevance to a broader patient population.

Validity determines the methodologic quality of the evidence, essentially considering how close the results correlate to potential 'truth' (particularly in the case of primary evidence). A validity assessment considers the robustness of the methods used to carry out the research, which will vary according to the type of research performed (e.g. quantitative, qualitative, mixed-methods) and the question being asked.

The **strength** of the evidence is determined by a review of the results section, considering the significance of the findings and whether there is sufficient power within the data to draw conclusions. **Power** is the probability of observing a difference between groups in a sample when one is indeed present.[18]

Medical imaging investigations are a significant component of the diagnostic test landscape, with research into the accuracy of medical imaging investigations directly impacted by these reporting standards. A **diagnostic accuracy study** considers how well one or more test classifies a patient as having a target condition. This is not limited to the binary positive or negative diagnosis, but also can consider the test's ability to accurately stage the condition and/or monitor response to treatment (as dictated by the research question). The **index test** is the investigation under study, and it is compared to the **clinical reference** *standard*, which is the test considered the current best available method for evaluating the condition. A clinical reference standard may not necessarily be a **gold standard** – which is a test considered to be 'error-free'.

The **STARD** (Standards for Reporting of Diagnostic Accuracy Studies) guidelines were released in 2003 and updated in 2015, aiming to improve the transparency and accuracy of reporting diagnostic accuracy studies.[27] They were developed to address incomplete reporting of diagnostic accuracy studies, where essential parts of the study, including complete study protocols/methodologies, were not reported, hindering the ability to appraise the work. The guidelines have resulted in a small but statistically significant improvement in the overall quality of reporting diagnostic accuracy studies.

The STARD list of essential items for reporting diagnostic accuracy studies incorporates 30 items that should be included in every report.[27] The checklist aims to reduce bias and elevate data reporting beyond simple statistics (e.g. sensitivity and specificity). The heterogeneity of study populations, and even the individual contexts of the patient's healthcare journey should be considered when evaluating the accuracy of a diagnostic test.

The **QUADAS** (Quality Assessment of Diagnostic Accuracy Studies) tool was developed as a guide to help evaluate the risk of bias in diagnostic accuracy studies and assess their applicability to a broader population. It was designed more specifically to guide those conducting a systemic review; however, it can be used in the critical appraisal of diagnostic accuracy studies. It consists of four domains[28]:

- Patient selection
- Index test
- Reference Standard
- Flow and timing

Each of the four domains is assessed by a series of questions regarding signalling and risk of bias, and the patient selection, index test and reference standard domains are assessed for applicability.

The presentation of sensitivity and specificity data should be reviewed for studies evaluating diagnostic radiology studies. Sensitivity and specificity are impacted by the diagnostic threshold and can be impacted by the severity of cases included in the study population. The prevalence of disease in a population can impact the positive predictive value and negative predictive value of a test and, therefore, impact its applicability to other broader populations. If two diagnostic tests are being compared, the use of a ROC curve is an important inclusion.

For interventional or therapeutic studies, the hazard ratio, relative risk and attributable risk should be reviewed, as well as the number needed to treat.[24] Review of *P*-values and confidence intervals is also important to evaluate the potential impact of the intervention and the precision of the research's predictions.

When reviewing systematic reviews and meta-analyses, tools such as PRISMA, which are used to create the review, can equally be used in appraisal.[14,15] PRISMA provides a checklist of 27 items to appraise.

Step 4: Apply

In the fourth step of the appraisal, the results from the chosen article (or articles) are reviewed regarding:[24]

- The level of evidence of the article
- The internal and external validity
- The similarity of PICO of the article and that of the clinical question
- How the results relate to the original patient

For the review of diagnostic accuracy studies, the sensitivity and specificity and how they relate to the individual patient's diagnostic probability are considered. For interventional studies, the similarity of the study and local population should be examined to consider whether adjustments to the risk probability profiles and number needed to treat are required.

Step 5: Evaluate

The final stage of the appraisal consists of evaluating how the study's results could be applied to or alter local practice.[24] This process needs to be conducted with an appreciation of the rapidly growing and evolving nature of imaging technologies and an understanding that technology evolution will continue to impact clinical outcomes. Any limitations and gaps within the available literature should also be discussed at this stage.

BOX 4.9   PRACTICE QUESTIONS

- Define evidence-based practice as it relates to clinical radiology.
- Outline the process of critically appraising a research paper.
- Describe how you would assess the validity of a research study, making reference to bias and the context of the research.

REFERENCES

1. National Health and Medical Research Council (NHMRC). *National Statement on Ethical Conduct in Human Research 2023.* Canberra: National Health and Medical Research Council, Commonwealth of Australia, 2023.
2. National Institutes of Health. Guiding principles for ethical research: Pursuing potential research participants protections. *National Institutes of Health Website*, https://www.nih.gov/health-information/nih-clinical-research-trials-you/guiding-principles-ethical-research (2016, accessed 6 September 2024).
3. Armond ACV, Cobey KD, Moher D. Key concepts in clinical epidemiology: Research integrity definitions and challenges. *Journal of Clinical Epidemiology* 2024; *171*: 111367.
4. Sica GT. Bias in research studies. *Radiology* 2006; *238*: 780–789.
5. The University of Sydney. *Academic Integrity.* The University of Sydney, https://www.sydney.edu.au/students/academic-integrity/breaches.html (2024, accessed 6 September 2024).

6. Fossey E, Harvey C, McDermott F, et al. Understanding and evaluating qualitative research. *Australian & New Zealand Journal of Psychiatry* 2002; *36*: 717–732.

7. Shedlock A. 8 Examples of qualitative research. *Greenbook*, https://www.greenbook.org/insights/qualitative-market-research/8-examples-of-qualitative-research (2024, accessed 5 September 2024).

8. Sale JEM, Lohfeld LH, Brazil K. Revisiting the quantitative-qualitative debate: implications for mixed-methods research. *Quality and Quantity*, 2002; *36*: 43–53.

9. University of Oxford: Centre for Evidence-Based Medicine. *Study Designs*, https://www.cebm.ox.ac.uk/resources/ebm-tools/study-designs (2024, accessed 5 September 2024).

10. Stolberg HO, Norman G, Trop I. Randomized controlled trials. *American Journal of Roentgenology* 2004; *183*: 1539–1544.

11. Blackmore CC, Cummings P. Observational studies in radiology. *American Journal of Roentgenology* 2004; *183*: 1203–1208.

12. McInnes MDF, Bossuyt PMM. Pitfalls of systematic reviews and meta-analyses in imaging research. *Radiology* 2015; *277*: 13–21.

13. Higgins JPT, Thomas J, Chandler J, et al. *Cochrane Handbook for Systematic Reviews of Interventions.* 2nd ed. Hoboken, NJ: The Cochrane Collaboration and John Wiley & Sons Ltd., (2019).

14. Page MJ, McKenzie JE, Bossuyt PM, et al. The PRISMA 2020 statement: An updated guideline for reporting systematic reviews. *The BMJ 372*: 1–9.

15. PRISMA. Preferred Reporting Items for Systematic reviews and Meta-Analyses (PRISMA) website, https://www.prisma-statement.org/ (2024, accessed 5 September 2024).

16. Postgraduate Research - The University of Sydney. How to write a research proposal. *The University of Sydney*, https://www.sydney.edu.au/study/applying/how-to-apply/postgraduate-research/how-to-write-a-research-proposal-for-a-strong-phd-application.html (2024, accessed 6 September 2024).

17. Atzen SL. Top 10 tips for writing materials and methods in radiology: A brief guide for authors. *Radiology* 2024; *310*: 1–5.

18. Anvari A, Halpern EF, Samir AE. Statistics 101 for radiologists. *Radiographics* 2015; *35*: 1789–1801.

19. Weinstein S, Obuchowski NA, Lieber ML. Clinical evaluation of diagnostic tests. *American Journal of Roentgenology* 2005; *184*: 14–19.

20. Obuchowski NA. ROC analysis. *American Journal of Roentgenology* 2005; *184*: 364–372.

21. Lavelle LP, Dunne RM, Carroll AG, et al. Evidence-based practice of radiology. *Radiographics* 2015; *35*: 1802–1813.

22. Evidence-Based Medicine Working Group. Evidence-based medicine: A new approach to teaching the practice of medicine. *JAMA* 1992; *268*: 2420–2425.

23. Burns PB, Rohrich RJ, Chung KC. The levels of evidence and their role in evidence-based medicine. *Plastic and Reconstructive Surgery* 2011; *128*: 305–310.

24. Sadigh G, Parker R, Kelly AM, et al. How to write a critically appraised topic (CAT). *Academic Radiology* 2012; *19*: 872–888.

25. DiCenso A, Bayley L, Haynes B. Accessing pre-appraised evidence: Fine-tuning the 5S model into a 6S model. *Evidence-Based Nursing* 2009; *12*: 99–101.

26. McMaster University. *Resources for Evidence-Based Practice: The 6S Pyramid.* Health Sciences Library: Guides & Tutorials, https://hslmcmaster.libguides.com/ebm/6s-pyramid (2024, accessed 29 August 2024).

27. Bossuyt PM, Reitsma JB, Bruns DE, et al. STARD 2015: An updated list of essential items for reporting diagnostic accuracy studies1. *Radiology* 2015; *277*: 826–832.

28. University of Bristol. *QUADAS.* University of Bristol: Population Health Sciences, https://www.bristol.ac.uk/population-health-sciences/projects/quadas/quadas-2/ (accessed 5 September 2024).

Cultural Safety, Advocacy and Emerging Technology

5

At the outset of this chapter, I want to acknowledge that I am a white Australian woman. This chapter considers some sensitive but extremely important topics, such as equity in healthcare, cultural safety and healthcare provision to First Peoples. It is difficult to do justice to the depth of these topics within the scope of a review book, and I am in no way able to speak on behalf of the personal experiences of these groups. I do aim to provide definitions and a framework for you to build your knowledge through other resources and personal experience. The references throughout this chapter cite expansive articles, guidelines, and websites. I warmly encourage to you explore them if you are interested in expanding your knowledge.

PRINCIPLES OF EQUITY AND CULTURAL SAFETY IN HEALTHCARE

Equity in healthcare

The World Health Organization defines **equity** as

> the absence of unfair, avoidable or remediable differences among groups of people, whether those groups are defined socially, economically, demographically, or geographically or by other dimensions of inequality (e.g. sex, gender, ethnicity, disability, or sexual orientation). Health equity is achieved when everyone can attain their full potential for health and wellbeing.[1]

DOI: 10.1201/9781003466529-5

Equity differs from **equality**, which is when the division of resources is equal among a group of people. Equality does not consider the inherent differences in a population or the fact that some individuals may be in a position of disadvantage. Equity considers that resources should be allocated based on need in the interest of giving each member of the group the opportunity of an equal outcome.

Healthcare equity is impacted by complex social, financial and cultural factors, and can be affected by both conscious and unconscious biases. Healthcare disparities are seen as differences in the incidence and prevalence of certain conditions in sub-groups of the population compared to a broader population average. These differences are often the result of healthcare inequity, and may be secondary to issues with access to quality healthcare, education or employment, or differences in how healthcare professionals treat the population.[2]

Conscious and unconscious bias

Bias is present when there is a prejudice towards or against a person or group of people in a manner considered unfair. Bias can be either conscious or unconscious.

Conscious bias, also known as explicit bias, is a bias that we and those around us are aware of. Conscious bias includes deliberate prejudice and discriminatory practices based on factors such as ethnicity, gender, sexuality or disability.

Unconscious bias, also known as implicit bias, can be more insidious. Social and cultural stereotypes can form outside of a person's conscious awareness, often meaning they do not realise they possess the bias at all. Addressing unconscious bias is challenging for this reason, and broaching the issue has the potential to cause division and offence.

Unconscious bias can influence healthcare at all levels, from the individual to the organisational level to the whole population. At the individual level, unconscious bias can impact the attitudes and perceptions the healthcare provider holds about those around them and themselves. At an organisational level, unconscious bias can affect hiring policies, the distribution of roles and responsibilities, and healthcare provision. At a population-based level, unconscious bias can result in healthcare inequity if left unchecked.

Principles of cultural safety

Cultural safety is an overarching paradigm encompassing and going beyond cultural awareness, sensitivity, respect and competence. The meaning of cultural safety is variable, and there is no universally agreed-upon definition.

Cultural awareness involves acknowledging of the difference between groups of people based on culture and considering how that impacts the attitudes and behaviours of ourselves and others.[3]

Cultural sensitivity and cultural respect are similar concepts. **Cultural sensitivity** is the awareness of cultural differences and the need to respect these differences.[3] **Cultural respect** is defined as the recognition, protection and continued advancement of the inherent rights, cultures and traditions of a particular culture.[4]

Cultural safety goes beyond this, bringing these values into practice to create an environment in which people of all cultures feel safe, valued, respected, and included. For this to be achieved, individuals and organisations need to be open-minded and adaptable in their beliefs and appreciation of cultures other than their own.

Cultural competence is exercised when a clinician 'has the attitudes, skills and knowledge needed to function effectively and respectfully when working with and treating people of different cultural backgrounds'.[5] While important, this metric alone is insufficient to produce a culturally safe environment for all patients. Some authors have also raised concerns that the concept of cultural competence erroneously implies a static threshold for proficiency and may pose a barrier to ongoing learning and reflection.[6]

Institutional racism (also known as systemic racism) is when racism and racial biases are ingrained into the policies and practices of an entire organisation or society. This results in a system that perpetuates discrimination of one or more social, ethnic or cultural groups to the advantage of others. In healthcare, institutional racism can include disproportionate or discriminatory control of, and access to, information and power imbalances between healthcare workers and patients. Institutional racism has been identified as a major contributor to the health gap between First Peoples and non-Indigenous people in Australia and New Zealand and between ethnic and racial minority groups in the USA and the UK (and more broadly around the world).[7]

Cultural safety is paramount in providing equitable healthcare to First Peoples worldwide. In Australia, the Australian Healthcare Practitioners Regulatory Association (AHPRA) addresses cultural safety in Aboriginal and Torres Strait Islander people as a non-negotiable component of healthcare provision. AHPRA defines cultural safety 'as the individual and institutional knowledge, skills, attitudes and competencies needed to deliver optimal health care for Aboriginal and Torres Strait Islander Peoples.'[8] The policy also affirms that what constitutes cultural safety is to be determined by the Aboriginal and Torres Strait Islander people themselves.

In Aotearoa New Zealand, standards of practice and legislation require health professionals to provide culturally safe care, including integrating the principles of Te Tiriti o Waitangi (The Treaty of Waitangi) into practice.[9]

Culturally safe practice requires clinicians and other healthcare providers to engage in continued reflection and improvement across their practice. This includes examining the impact of one's culture on clinical interactions and the provision of healthcare services. Through this, the practitioner needs to acknowledge and address their own unconscious biases, attitudes, assumptions, prejudices and characteristics, which may impact the quality of care they provide to different groups of patients.[3]

Acknowledging the impact of cultural safety and institutional racism on healthcare (Australia & New Zealand)

In both Australia and New Zealand, there are striking healthcare discrepancies between the health and life expectancy of First Peoples compared to non-Indigenous people.

In New Zealand, the life expectancy of Māori people is, on average, 7.3 years less than their non-Indigenous counterparts.[6] The inequities extend to health outcomes, with Māori people having the overall poorest health quality of any ethnic group in New Zealand.

The 2020 *Closing the Gap* report found that the Aboriginal and Torres Strait Islander people of Australia have similar poor comparative health outcomes.[10] On average, Aboriginal and Torres Strait Islander men have a life expectancy of 8.6 years less than non-Indigenous men. The life expectancy of Indigenous women was 7.8 years less on average compared to non-Indigenous Australian women. The mortality rate in Aboriginal and Torres Strait Islander children was double that of the rest of the population.

Approximately half of the discrepancy in health outcomes between Indigenous and non-Indigenous Australians has been attributed to the social determinants of health and risk factors, with the other half linked with racism (interpersonal and institutional) and the effects of intergenerational trauma.[7]

Intergenerational trauma is when the impact of a significant traumatic event is passed on from one generation to the next. In Australia, the effects of intergenerational trauma are seen in the descendants of the Stolen Generations.

The Stolen Generations refer to a period between approximately 1905 and the 1970s when government policies facilitated the forced removal of mixed-race Aboriginal children from their families. The number of children removed is unknown, but is thought to be well over 100,000. Children were removed under the guise of 'resocialisation' as part of deliberate racist assimilation policies and placed under the care of government-controlled facilities or adoptive white families. Removed children were separated from their families, culture and land, with many exposed to abuse and neglect.[11] The Australian Government offered a formal apology to the Stolen Generations in 2008.

Ongoing social, economic and health disparities are seen in the people of the Stolen Generations and their descendants, who have overall decreased health and well-being outcomes compared to the general population and other Indigenous people.[11,12] The Healing Foundation writes:

> *Stolen Generations survivors might also pass on the impacts of institutionalisation, finding it difficult to know how to nurture their children because they were denied the opportunity to be nurtured themselves.*[11]

Addressing cultural safety, institutional racism and health equity

An inclusive workplace and patient-care culture is the foundation for promoting cultural safety in radiology practice. Department leaders and managers who encourage and model culturally safe behaviours and practices are also integral to the process.

An inclusive culture can be developed by:[13]

- Minimising intentional and unintentional microaggressions in ourselves and recognising and calling out the behaviour in others

- Recognising and addressing unconscious bias in recruitment, leadership pathways, research involvement and other administrative processes
- Encouraging diversity, equity and inclusion across all aspects of the workplace and implementing strategies to promote this e.g. mentorship programs

Addressing the more insidious issue of institutional racism in medical imaging practice and healthcare more broadly is complex and best targeted with a top-down approach. While there is a role for targeted education and resource provision for staff, this needs to be supported by governments, organisations and leaders within healthcare institutions. Fundamentally, doctors and other health providers should know and demonstrate an understanding of Indigenous rights and the issues that relate to their health and health equity.[14]

Strategies may include:[7,14]

- Revision of policies and redistribution of political power in governments and organisations to address disparities and remove embedded racism
- Specifically writing First Peoples into law, legislation and policy
- Reevaluating the balance of power between healthcare providers and patients, with a greater focus on cultural identity and social needs/priorities
- Funding redistribution towards Indigenous and/or minority initiatives (developed in line with culturally safe and inclusive practices)
- Ensuring there is an First Peoples' voice on representative and advisory boards and within healthcare leadership teams
- Incorporating models of health that are specific to the First Peoples, focusing on person-centred care but incorporating cultural priorities and identity

Organisational leaders can promote cultural safety and target institutional racism though:[7]

- Ensuring recruitment and hiring practices are inclusive and free from cultural bias
- Modelling and enforcing the principles of diversity, equity and inclusion
- Creating and supporting quality improvement initiatives aimed at targeting institutional racism and cultural competency

Cultural support staff

Cultural support workers and teams exist across health services to assist patients and staff. The primary role of a **cultural support worker** is the provision of cultural support and guidance to patients and their families and community, and healthcare staff to provide culturally appropriate care.[15] Cultural support workers can assist with bridging the gap between patients and those caring for them by ensuring cultural beliefs are incorporated, cultural and linguistic divides are acknowledged and addressed, and the autonomy of person-centred care is maintained.

Cultural support staff provide guidance and resources to facilitate culturally safe work practices and healthcare provision for health professionals. This may be through establishing connections with Indigenous and other cultural groups, mentorship and support programs, or specific awareness and educational initiatives.

For patients specifically, cultural support workers can provide psychological and emotional support as they navigate health services. Connecting with someone with shared cultural backgrounds and experiences can provide a safe space for patients and result in a more positive healthcare experience.[15]

Communication and cultural safety

One of the cornerstones of person-centred care is the shared understanding between the healthcare provider and the patient. This shared understanding is forged through effective communication; however, it hinges on the clinician's ability to bridge gaps in knowledge and trust. If a shared understanding cannot be reached, communication breaks down, and the quality of care is compromised.

A qualitative study, by Cass and colleagues,[16] found that shared understanding was only rarely achieved between healthcare staff and the Aboriginal patients attending a dialysis unit in remote Australia. Factors found to impact the quality of communication included:

- Lack of patient autonomy over the circumstances of health interactions, including in which language they were conducted, the time and the place the consultation took place, and the agenda or content discussed
- A dominance of Western discourse over the patient's cultural discourse, leading to a linguistic disconnect
- Healthcare providers determining whether an interpreter was required on behalf of the patient rather than allowing the patient to choose
- Patient's reluctance to answer medical questions truthfully out of politeness i.e. saying what they believe the clinician wants to hear
- Medical best-practice perceptions dominating and overcoming the social and cultural needs of the patient (e.g. geographical, financial and community priorities)
- Absence of resources and opportunities aimed at bridging the gap and reaching a shared understanding
- Health literacy inequities, especially with regard to complex medical conditions and procedures
- Low levels of staff engaging with resources and training in intercultural communication despite them being available and accessible

Many, if not all, of these impacts can be applied to medical imaging practice, particularly those related to financial, social and geographic inequity, accessible communication and provision of resources and training.

The study also found that describing risk as a percentage (as in traditional Western discourse) was poorly understood in some Aboriginal patients, as the concept was not commonplace. Radiologists may need to alter their explanations to convey procedural risk better to reach a shared understanding so that the patient can safely and legally provide informed consent.

Finally, Aboriginal patients highly value the 'talk' aspect of the consultation, when health practitioners take the time to talk to the patients at their level and on their terms. The process serves to mediate power differentials between the patient and the provider, leading to a greater chance of fostering trust and reaching a shared understanding.[17] This is linked to greater engagement and positive healthcare experiences and outcomes.

BOX 5.1   PRACTICE QUESTIONS

- Define cultural safety and describe how it relates to safe and effective clinical radiology practice.
- Define conscious and unconscious bias, considering how they may relate to clinical radiology practice.
- Discuss how the history of Aboriginal and Torres Strait Islander peoples or Māori and Pacific peoples may impact engagement with health services.
- Describe the role of cultural support staff (e.g. an Aboriginal Liaison Officer) in the healthcare of patients from minority cultural backgrounds.

SERVICE PROVISION TO VULNERABLE COMMUNITIES

Social determinants of health

Social determinants of health are non-medical circumstances that impact health outcomes. These include personal factors such as where someone was born, where they live, and how old they are, as well as broader systems and forces that influence and shape their daily lives. The social determinants have a wide-ranging impact on the health outcomes of all people, both positive and negative.

The World Health Organization (WHO) estimates that between a third and a half of health outcomes are influenced by the social determinants of health, which can be classified as related to:[18]

- Education
- Housing, amenities and living environments
- Early childhood development

- Social inclusion and exposure to discrimination
- Food insecurity
- Structural conflict
- Job security and employment/unemployment
- Working environment and conditions
- Access to affordable, quality healthcare

Addressing these factors is essential in working towards health equity and improving population outcomes. For patients accessing radiology services, social determinants of health can be mitigated by several strategies, including:[19]

- Mitigation of imaging costs
- Advocacy across platforms related to imaging availability, access and cost subsidisation
- Ensuring access to interpreter services and provision of culturally and linguistically appropriate resources
- Initiatives to improve health literacy
- Services to assist with healthcare navigation and cultural support
- Establishment or extension of imaging services to regional or marginalised communities

Healthcare inequity & barriers for rural and remote populations

Australians living in rural and remote communities are more likely to have reduced life expectancy, higher rates of injury and disease, and lower access to and engagement with healthcare compared with their counterparts in urban centres. For the patients themselves, healthcare inequity was driven by:[20]

- Geographic location and remoteness
- Financial and educational inequity
- Limited access to and availability of medical services
- Scarcity of medical experts
- Higher prevalence of risk factors for a range of health conditions

A review of the literature exploring access to healthcare for rural Australians identified several systematic barriers including:[20]

- Lack of informed leadership
- Inadequate clinical governance
- Limited awareness of current healthcare models
- Suboptimal workforce planning and resource allocation
- Incorrect risk perception
- Insufficient community engagement

Mobile medical imaging is one strategy for overcoming geographical and access barriers. This includes bringing service to remote communities or countries or those who may not be able to attend medical imaging practices, e.g. nursing home residents. Mobile radiology services have been utilised for over 100 years (including during World War I), but this service is growing with imaging technology and transport improvements. Modern radiology practices have been heavily reliant on transport and economic infrastructure to support the successful running of imaging machines, including the ability to staff and service the machines adequately.[21] In addition, stigma, social and cultural barriers can prevent members of some remote communities from attending medical imaging services if they are attached to large health services or hospitals. Other advantages of purpose-built mobile services are:

- Easier navigation through the service with simplified room layouts and less administrative steps
- Potential to raise awareness of health initiatives and screening programs
- Greater connection of communities with local healthcare providers and services
- Engagement with targeted health initiatives, e.g. mobile mammography units for breast cancer screening or mobile CT scanners for lung cancer screening

Barriers and inequities for people living with disabilities

For patients living with disabilities, the barriers to accessing healthcare can be amplified compared to others. These barriers extend beyond physical accessibility and hindrances of the environment, with challenges often overlapping. The Centre for Disease Control (CDC) divides these barriers into:[22]

- **Attitudinal:** lack of awareness of the needs of people with disabilities, stereotypes, stigma
- **Communication:** breakdown or inability to adequately communicate with persons with specific disabilities such as visual, auditory or cognitive impairment
- **Physical:** obstacles to mobility and/or access e.g. difficulty accessing mammography equipment for patients unable to stand
- **Policy:** lack of awareness or enforcement of laws to prevent discrimination, provision of accommodation or accessible options, or denial of benefits
- **Programmatic:** inconvenient scheduling or time allocation, poor knowledge, communication and attitudes among providers
- **Social:** inequities in the social determinants of health e.g. lower employment rates, lower high school graduation rates, lower average income, higher risk of exposure to violence and other forms of abuse
- **Transportation:** lack of access to convenient and cost-effective transport, dependent on the specific nature of the disability

Improving access to imaging services for First Peoples

Social determinants of health and health equity for First Peoples and communities are discussed in more depth in *Chapter 5: Principles of equity and cultural safety in healthcare*. Specific enablers of access to quality health and medical imaging services for Indigenous people and communities can include:[23]

- Improved coordination of healthcare and medical imaging services
- Better communication between imaging staff and patients
- Fostering trust in medical services and exercising cultural safety and inclusivity
- Emphasising the importance of allowing patients and their community to express their health needs
- Provision of reliable, affordable and sustainable imaging services
- Maximising geographic and transport availability

BOX 5.2   PRACTICE QUESTIONS

- List three barriers to accessing quality medical imaging care, giving an example of how each could impact engagement with radiology services.
- Describe an evidence-based radiology service or resource which could be used to assist communities in need.
- Outline the importance of clinical radiologists engaging with consumer advocacy groups.

GENDER DIVERSITY IN CLINICAL RADIOLOGY

Gender inequality amongst radiologist workforces and subspecialties

In most radiology workforces worldwide, men outnumber women, with women accounting for approximately one-third of the global radiologist workforce. In Australia and New Zealand, approximately 30% of radiologists and 35% of training radiologists are women – despite women accounting for nearly half of Australian doctors.[24]

The benefits of gender diversity in medical imaging and other clinical teams include:[25]

- Greater innovation and creativity
- Fostering of inclusive culture
- Improved patient care and decision-making

Gender discrepancies are more pronounced in some subspecialties. Women are most under-represented in interventional radiology, interventional neuroradiology, musculoskeletal imaging and emergency radiology. In the United States, when the 48 largest specialty training programs are ranked by gender diversity, diagnostic radiology is 41st and interventional radiology 47th (second last).[26] In comparison, women are over-represented in breast and obstetrics/gynaecology imaging, which have traditionally been considered more 'female-friendly'.[24]

Potential contributors to the lack of gender diversity in radiology include:[27]

- Unconscious bias influencing recruitment and hiring processes
- Relative scarcity and lack of visibility of women role models and mentors
- Lack of exposure during medical training and junior doctor years
- Perceived lack of patient contact
- Lack of inclination towards physics and computing/digital health

Gender diversity in radiology leadership

Gender inequity is commonly observed to be more pronounced within representative leadership and senior academic faculty, with the proportions of women in these roles lagging behind the already disproportionate gender imbalance in the workforce. Significant improvements have occurred over the last few decades; however, addressing gender diversity among higher levels of leadership is an ongoing issue.

It is a misconception that gender equity in leadership will occur organically, eventually reflecting improvements in gender diversity in the broader workforce. However, this is rarely seen to be the case. Targeted initiatives are usually required to tackle a range of social, organisational, and political factors. Improvements have been shown in RSNA (Radiological Society of North America) representative membership, with gender parity now seen in committee chairs.[26] As of 2023, men still outnumber women on the RSNA Board.

The causes of a lack of gender diversity in representative leadership are complex and often overlapping. They include:[25]

- Unconscious bias surrounding the capability, credibility and capacity of current and potential women leaders
- Challenges related to work–life integration, particularly with regard to the expectation of women to take on carer roles in the home
- Relative sparsity of women role models and mentors
- Disproportionate loss of women from leadership development and senior management pathways ('leaky pipeline')
- Second-generation bias written into policies and guidelines or ingrained within an organisation or community's culture

The **leaky pipeline** metaphor is used to help model the unequal loss of women from leadership pathways compared to their male contemporaries. The percentage of women declines the further you move along the pipeline, from medical school through the radiology workforce and into leadership positions (Figure 5.1). Once a radiologist has left the leadership pipeline, it can be difficult for them to re-enter again.

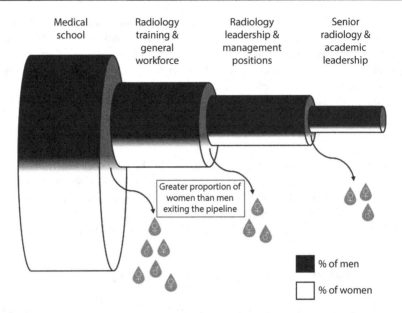

FIGURE 5.1   The 'leaky pipeline' in radiology leadership. Adapted from Weigel et al.[28]

Improving gender diversity in radiology leadership requires initiatives addressed at individual, institutional and organisational levels. For individual radiologists, recognising and challenging unconscious bias about gender is a good first step. These biases not only impact our perception of others but can also impact how women see themselves. For example, a woman is more likely to take herself out of the running for a leadership role due to negative self-perceptions or her suitability. Organisations and department leadership need to acknowledge issues with gender diversity, model inclusive practices and demonstrate strong leadership commitment to change.

Some solutions that have been proposed to improve gender diversity in radiology leadership include:[25]

- Initiatives to empower and connect women e.g. societies, events, awards
- Establishment of subcommittees and working parties to address gender inequity in leadership
- Resource development & provision of unconscious bias training
- Provision of scholarships and additional training to women interested in leadership
- Initiatives to re-engage mid-career radiologists with leadership development pathways
- Gender targets for committee or interview panel composition

---

BOX 5.3   PRACTICE QUESTION

- Outline the status of gender diversity in the radiology workforce and list three strategies that could be implemented to address it.

ARTIFICIAL INTELLIGENCE (AI) AND EMERGING TECHNOLOGIES

Principles of AI and machine learning

Artificial intelligence (AI) encompasses technology developed to simulate human intelligence and advanced functions in computers and machines. AI functions include learning, problem-solving, visual perception, translation, and comprehensive and creative applications such as image and music generation and modification.

Machine learning is a subset of AI. Whereas AI can be simplified as computers and machines simulating human functions, machine learning can be considered as teaching a computer to perform a specific task as accurately as possible. **Machine learning** is defined as a 'method of data science that provides computers with the ability to learn without being programmed with explicit rules'.[29] Machine learning analyses large datasets to find patterns and relationships between the data without any specific rules or programming. Continuous iterative improvement allows the creation of algorithms to learn and make predictions in future datasets.

There are three main subtypes of machine learning: supervised, unsupervised and reinforced learning (Table 5.1). Supervised and unsupervised machine learning can be used together, with a reinforced learning feedback loop. **Ground truth** is information known to be true in the real world that is used to calibrate a machine learning algorithm.

One application of machine learning is the creation of neural networks. **Neural networks** are machine learning programs or models that mimic the biological connectivity and decision capacity of the human brain. Data entered into the network is processed by engaging interconnected nodes, with the nodes passing data between each other. These nodes within the network act similarly to neurons, with links between them simulating biological synapses.

Neural networks have three layers: an input layer, a 'hidden' layer and an output layer. Inputs may include images or text. The hidden layer often consists of multiple layers determined by the complexity of the task or model. Adding more layers allows the neural network to engage in more sophisticated predictions. Deep learning requires multiple hidden layers due to the task's inherent complexity.

TABLE 5.1   Subtypes of machine learning.

Supervised	• Data labels given to the algorithm in the training phase • Expected outputs labelled by human experts (ground truth) • Goal is to learn a general rule mapping inputs to outputs
Unsupervised	• No data labels provided to the algorithm • Goal is to find hidden patterns and structures within the data, and then separate the data into groups
Reinforced learning	• Computing tasks performed in a dynamic environment • Feedback provided to the algorithm • Positive and negative reinforcement guide learning

Adapted from Choy et al.[29]

Deep learning is a subset of machine learning which uses multi-level neural networks. These progressively extract higher-level information from the inputs and recognise more complex patterns. Deep learning models are considered more autonomous and accurate than traditional or simplified machine learning algorithms. There are broad applications for deep learning algorithms, including image recognition and natural language processing.

Natural language processing is a section of AI considering computer interpretation of human language. Voice recognition, widely used by radiologists, is an application of this technology. Emerging models that examine the processing and generation of the written report utilise natural language processing.

Radiomics is 'a quantitative approach to medical imaging, which aims at enhancing the existing data available to clinicians by means of advanced mathematical analysis'.[30] AI algorithms analyse numeric data from medical images (e.g. intensity measurements and relationships between pixels) to discern textural differences. These models aim to provide decision support and help detect hidden patterns and diagnoses imperceptible to the radiologist's eye.

Applications of machine learning and AI in radiology

AI applications have been integrated into routine radiology for over a decade. Examples include computer-aided detection (CAD) software to assist in interpreting breast MRI or oncology studies, computer-aided image analysis software to analyse CT perfusion studies investigating acute stroke and voice recognition software. New applications are constantly emerging, potentially impacting all aspects of medical imaging practice (Table 5.2).

TABLE 5.2　Examples of current and potential applications of AI in medical imaging[29,31–33]

Administration & pre-arrival	• Booking & scheduling • Patient screening & questionnaires	• Study protocolling • Billing/financials
Study acquisition & image processing	• Acquisition automation • Image data processing • Radiation dose reduction • Decreased scanning time (MRI) • Image analytics	• Post-processing automation e.g. reconstructions, segmentation • Image quality improvement/enhancement
Image review	• Work list optimisation and triage • Image display/hanging protocols • Automated measurements	• Case pre-analysis & information extraction including findings detection +/- interpretation • Lesion tracking
Reporting	• Speech recognition and translation • Report text applications e.g. creation, template integration, editing, language level adjustment	• Report summary and critical finding detection/ highlighting • Clinical decision support
Quality assurance, data management & research	• Radiation dose estimation • Radiology reporting and analytics • Data integration and analysis (multiple studies, clinical information, radiomics)	• Data storage • Image-based search engine e.g. education, comparison cases • Population health integration and research

Intrinsic and data challenges related to AI in imaging

Intrinsic challenges in AI relate to the capability of the technology and the science surrounding it. Examples of intrinsic challenges include:[31]

- Establishment and definitions of 'truth'
- Applicability of models to broader populations
- Speed of processing
- Tolerance of protocols

Large data sets are required to train machine learning algorithms and neural networks In imaging, that means that algorithms require access to large sets of patient images. To source these large data sets, ethical considerations and institutional barriers to consider include:[29,31,33]

- Maintenance of patient confidentiality around image use and integration of clinical data
- Appropriateness of the use of patient data beyond their images e.g. for clinical integration
- Data management, security and storage
- Proprietary restrictions (medico-legal) and institutional barriers preventing amalgamation of images across practices and institutions

For applications already developed and approved for clinical use, there can be barriers to integrating the software into existing reporting systems and imaging technologies. If significant system upgrades are required, there may be institutional and staff resistance and potentially higher financial costs at the outset.

Circumstantial challenges related to AI in imaging

Circumstantial challenges refer to the human and societal behavioural considerations regarding the integration and use of AI technologies in medical imaging, and society more broadly.[31] Specific challenges and barriers include:

- Concerns over the 'replacement' of the radiology workforce
- Clinician trust in the technology
- Regulatory body approval of AI technologies for use in healthcare
- Shortage of AI and machine learning-trained clinicians to participate in research

The early discourse surrounding AI's emerging role in medical imaging raised concerns that the technology would quickly replace the radiologist workforce. This conversation has evolved and now focuses on successfully integrating clinical practice with AI tools.

Humans and AI have the potential to work well together to improve patient care and the betterment of medical imaging as a discipline. Both offer (or have the potential to offer) different strengths in the clinical assessment, problem-solving and management processes.[32] There is also the potential for enhanced delivery of precision medicine and integration with radiogenomics.[29]

Current AI applications (which have a narrow task focus rather than a broad general intelligence) have the potential to offer more precise imaging interpretation, more efficiently work through larger data sets, and find patterns that would have been otherwise hidden. Humans, in comparison, can make inferences from comparatively smaller amounts of data and can contextualise information better to suit local practice and specific patients. In addition, humans can offer superior patient communication and better consider relationships and the broader patient context.[32]

For clinicians to work effectively with AI applications, they need to be able to trust their outputs. This includes ensuring that the data is accurate and that patient safety and confidentiality are maintained.[33] This links to the intrinsic challenge of generalisability of machine learning models and applications, noting that the results from training on a certain data set may not apply to the population more broadly or to smaller population subsets.

'Black Box' refers to the issue of humans being unable to see how deep learning systems make decisions. This can lead to uncertainty surrounding the technology or mistrust. Strategies to combat this include greater education and transparency around the use of the AI application e.g. using annotated case sets to help educate users as to the rationale for the system's decisions.[34]

While AI algorithms can potentially increase diagnostic accuracy, this must be balanced against the risk of over diagnosing certain conditions.[33] Overdiagnosis of certain conditions (e.g. thyroid nodules and adrenal adenomas) can harm patients through unnecessary additional imaging and follow-up studies. Integrating AI results with clinician input can mediate this risk.

As AI technologies are unlike traditional medical devices and software packages, there have been concerns regarding regulatory processes and approvals of AI applications as they move into clinical practice. Note that many applications have already been approved for and are in use in clinical practice. The risks and benefits of some characteristics of AI applications are poorly understood; for example, the implications of continual iterative learning of an application already deployed in clinical settings.[35]

Considerations when adapting to new technologies

As radiology is inherently linked to technology, it is constantly innovating and changing by nature. For perspective, CT scans were only integrated into clinical practice in the 1970s, and MRI scanning was introduced in the early 1980s. Positron emission tomography (PET) scans transitioned from research to clinical practice in the early 1990s, only gaining traction towards the turn of the century.[36] In those early days, it was grainy black-and-white data only, and it was another decade before modern PET/CT cameras, as we knew them, were truly integrated into patient care. Australian and New Zealand radiology fellowship exam candidates were examined on printed film until 2020 when COVID-19 necessitated electronic delivery of the oral exam for the first time.

While change is expected, it brings a range of challenges for the radiologists and the broader medical imaging department. Some examples are outlined in Figure 5.2.

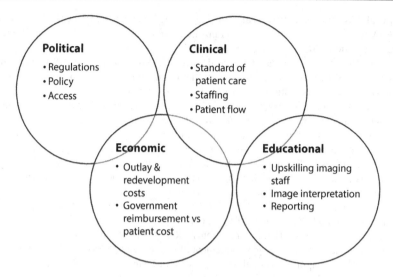

FIGURE 5.2   Some examples of challenges faced by radiologists and imaging departments during the introduction of new technologies.

When new technologies are introduced, the radiologist must be open and willing to learn how to use them safely and effectively. This applies to something as grand as a new imaging modality or as small as a new image software package. Ideally, the department and/or vendor will provide educational resources and support to assist individual radiologists and other staff in familiarising themselves with the system. Only when staff are adequately trained should their new skills and knowledge be utilised for clinical care.

BOX 5.4   PRACTICE QUESTIONS

- Discuss the current use of an AI application in medical imaging practice and explain how it positively impacts patient care.
- Outline some challenges which may be encountered when integrating a new AI system into a medical imaging workflow.
- Discuss some challenges a radiology department may face when implementing a new software package into diagnostic reporting. How may these be overcome?

REFERENCES

1. World Health Organization. *Health Equity*. World Health Organization, https://www.who.int/health-topics/health-equity (2024, accessed 6 September 2024).
2. Americo L, Ramjit A, Wu M, et al. Health care disparities in radiology: A primer for resident education. *Current Problems in Diagnostic Radiology* 2019; *48*: 108–110.

3. Royal Australian and New Zealand College of Radiologists (RANZCR). Cultural safety. *RANZCR Website*, https://www.ranzcr.com/trainees/resources-and-support/trainees/cultural-safety (2024, accessed 6 September 2024).

4. NSW Government. What is cultural safety? *NSW Government: Safework*, https://www.safework.nsw.gov.au/safety-starts-here/our-aboriginal-program/culturally-safe-workplaces/what-is-cultural-safety (2024, accessed 6 September 2024).

5. Te Tahu Hauora - Health Quality & Safety Commission. Health literacy, equity, cultural safety and competence. *Te Tahu Hauora – Health Quality & Safety Commission*, https://www.hqsc.govt.nz/our-work/leadership-and-capability/kaiawhina-workforce/health-literacy-equity-cultural-safety-and-competence/ (2021, accessed 6 September 2024).

6. Curtis E, Jones R, Tipene-Leach D, et al. Why cultural safety rather than cultural competency is required to achieve health equity: A literature review and recommended definition. *International Journal for Equity in Health* 2019; *18*: 1–17.

7. Bourke CJ, Marrie H, Marrie A. Transforming institutional racism at an Australian hospital. *Australian Health Review* 2018; *43*: 611–618.

8. AHPRA - Australian Health Practitioners Regulatory Agency. Aboriginal and Torres Strait Islander Health Strategy – Statement of Intent. *AHPRA Website*, https://www.ahpra.gov.au/About-Ahpra/Aboriginal-and-Torres-Strait-Islander-Health-Strategy/Statement-of-intent.aspx (2023, accessed 6 September 2024).

9. Te Whatu Ora (Health New Zealand). Cultural support for staff. *Te Whatu Ora (Health New Zealand) Website*, https://www.waikatodhb.health.nz/learning-and-research/learning/cultural-support-for-staff/ (2024, accessed 27 September 2024).

10. Australian Government. *Closing the Gap: Report 2020*. Canberra, https://ctgreport.niaa.gov.au/ (2020, accessed 27 September 2024).

11. The Healing Foundation. *The Healing Foundation*. 2024, https://healingfoundation.org.au/ (accessed 27 September 2024).

12. Australian Institute of Health and Welfare. *Children Living in Households with Members of the Stolen Generations*. Canberra, https://www.aihw.gov.au/reports/indigenous-australians/children-living-in-households-with-members-of-the/summary (2019, accessed 27 September 2024).

13. Hennebry J, Debenedectis CM, Guzmán Pérez-Carrillo GJ, et al. Cultural competency in the radiology workplace. *In Practice*, https://arrsinpractice.org/radiology-workplace-cultural-competency/ (2022, accessed 27 September 2024).

14. Te Kaunihera Rata O Aotearoa (The Medical Council of New Zealand). *He Ara Hauora Māori: A Pathway to Māori Health Equity*. Wellington, New Zealand, https://www.mcnz.org.nz/assets/standards/6c2ece58e8/He-Ara-Hauora-Maori-A-Pathway-to-Maori-Health-Equity.pdf (October 2019, accessed 27 September 2024).

15. Goh M. Exploring the role of cultural support workers in the New Zealand healthcare setting. *Aotearoa New Zealand Social Work* 2018; *30*: 68–74.

16. Cass A, Lowell A, Christie M, et al. Sharing the true stories: Improving communication between Aboriginal patients and healthcare workers. *Medical Journal of Australia* 2002; *176*: 466–470.

17. Jennings W, Bond C, Hill PS. The power of talk and power in talk: A systematic review of Indigenous narratives of culturally safe healthcare communication. *Australian Journal of Primary Health* 2018; *24*: 109–115.

18. World Health Organization (WHO). Social determinants of health. *WHO Website*, https://www.who.int/health-topics/social-determinants-of-health (2024, accessed 28 September 2024).

19. Elmohr MM, Javed Z, Dubey P, et al. Social determinants of health framework to identify and reduce barriers to imaging in marginalized communities. *Radiology* 2024; *310*: e223097.

20. Baazeem M, Kruger E, Tennant M. Current status of tertiary healthcare services and its accessibility in rural and remote Australia: A systematic review. *Health Sciences Review* 2024; 100158.
21. Mollura DJ, England RW, Harvey SC, et al. Mobile strategies for global health radiology. *Radiology in Global Health: Strategies, Implementation, and Applications*. Cham: Springer; 2019; 283–307.
22. Centre for Disease Control (CDC). Disability barriers to inclusion. *CDC Website*, https://www.cdc.gov/ncbddd/disabilityandhealth/disability-barriers.htm (2024, accessed 28 September 2024).
23. Nolan-Isles D, Macniven R, Hunter K, et al. Enablers and barriers to accessing healthcare services for Aboriginal people in New South Wales, Australia. *International Journal of Environmental Research and Public Health* 2021; *18*: 3014.
24. Hayter CL, Ayesa SL. Female representation in radiology subspecialty interest groups in Australia and New Zealand. *Journal of Medical Imaging and Radiation Oncology* 2023; *67*: 162–169.
25. Ayesa SL, McEniery JC, Hill LS, et al. Navigating the glass labyrinth: Addressing gender diversity in Australian and New Zealand representative radiology leadership. *Journal of Medical Imaging and Radiation Oncology* 2023; *67*: 155–161.
26. Wang M, Yong-Hing C, Tomblinson C, et al. Diversity, equity, and inclusion in radiology: How far we have come in narrowing the gender gap. *RadioGraphics* 2024; *44*: e240033.
27. Jansen C, van Heerden X, Newell M. Women in radiology: Breaking the barriers of gender diversity: An opinion on the current literature. *European Journal of Radiology* *164*: 110863.
28. Weigel KS, Kubik-Huch RA, Gebhard C. Women in radiology: Why is the pipeline still leaking and how can we plug it? *Acta Radiologica* 2020; *61*: 743–748.
29. Choy G, Khalilzadeh O, Michalski M, et al. Current applications and future impact of machine learning in radiology. *Radiology* 2018; *288*: 318–328.
30. Van Timmeren JE, Cester D, Tanadini-Lang S, et al. Radiomics in medical imaging – 'how-to' guide and critical reflection. *Insights Imaging* 2020; *11*: 91.
31. Thrall JH, Li X, Li Q, et al. Artificial intelligence and machine learning in radiology: Opportunities, challenges, pitfalls, and criteria for success. *Journal of the American College of Radiology* 2018; *15*: 504–508.
32. Lakhani P, Prater AB, Hutson RK, et al. Machine learning in radiology: Applications beyond image interpretation. *Journal of the American College of Radiology* 2018; *15*: 350–359.
33. Wichmann JL, Willemink MJ, De Cecco CN. Artificial intelligence and machine learning in radiology: Current state and considerations for routine clinical implementation. *Investigative Radiology* 2020; *55*: 619–627.
34. Baselli G, Codari M, Sardanelli F. Opening the black box of machine learning in radiology: Can the proximity of annotated cases be a way? *European Radiology Experimental* 2020; *4*: 30.
35. Kohli M, Prevedello LM, Filice RW, et al. Implementing machine learning in radiology practice and research. *American Journal of Roentgenology* 2017; *208*: 754–760.
36. Ayesa SL, Murphy A. Positron emission tomography: Evolving modalities, radiopharmaceuticals and professional collaboration. *Journal of Medical Radiation Sciences* 2022; *69*: 415–418.

Advice for Applications and Exams

6

PREPARING FOR RADIOLOGY APPLICATIONS AND INTERVIEWS

To the junior doctors and medical students reading this: I am thrilled that you are here and interested in a career in radiology, nuclear medicine, or both. Medical imaging is a diverse specialty that is intellectually stimulating and constantly evolving, and I know that you will find a niche that suits your unique talents and interests.

In recent years, radiology training positions have become highly sought after and increasingly competitive, at least in my experience in Australia. This is partly due to the 'Medical Student Tsunami' (a term coined by then Australian Medical Students' Association president Teresa Cosgriff in the mid-2000s) and the increasing desirability of radiology as a specialty.

The range of subspecialties, the flexibility of working hours and days as a specialist, the integration with technology and the fulfilment that comes with providing a valued clinical service make radiology increasingly attractive. This increasing competitiveness should not discourage you, but rather motivate you to prepare yourself well for applications and interviews. Take a moment to start reflecting on why you are interested in radiology, why you think it is the right specialty for you and what you hope to achieve – it will come up again later.

Many prospective radiologists have approached me for information about my radiology and nuclear medicine journeys, seeking advice for applications and interviews and wanting to know about my experience working in medical imaging. You might have the same questions, so I have tried to answer them here. These are my experiences and opinions only, presented as suggestions rather than as a blueprint.

DOI: 10.1201/9781003466529-6

Why did I choose radiology and nuclear medicine?

If you had asked me in medical school whether I was considering radiology, I would have firmly answered 'No'. If you asked me if I were considering nuclear medicine, I would have asked you what nuclear medicine was. This speaks to the larger conversation about the image of both specialties. It seemed to me that radiologists worked in dark rooms, shied away from patient interaction, were never happy to see you and were almost all men. I couldn't see myself in the specialty and consequently dismissed it. Nuclear medicine did not factor into my medical education in a meaningful way. I had little understanding of how it was different to radiology (they are separate specialties in Australia) or how it fit into the care of my patients.

I tossed up different specialties but never really found one that fit well. By luck and circumstance, I ended up in a lecture during my intern year on head and neck radiology given by the incomparable Dr Robin Cassumbhoy. After that, there was no turning back.

In retrospect, my favourite parts of medicine were problem-solving and pattern recognition. I thought anatomy wasn't my strong suit and would be relieved whenever the CT slice replaced the cadaveric dissection. To me, it just made more sense. I went to physics camp when I was in high school. I loved working with computers and images and best expressed myself through the written word. All the signs were there, really.

I found nuclear medicine after a friend and I teamed up to study together for the anatomy component of the radiology exam. He was working in nuclear medicine as a junior doctor and loved it. We started studying together in his department, and I got to know some doctors there simply by being around. I had a unique situation: I was half a year behind my resident cohort as I had taken maternity leave at the start of the internship. I couldn't apply to radiology, but I was still looking for imaging experience. I applied for the nuclear medicine senior resident job for the next year and managed to land it. I wasn't their first choice, mind you: I was pulled off the eligibility list after an interview faux pas of my own.

I always said that the nuclear medicine senior resident job was the best I ever had. This remains true today, even though I now work as a consultant in the same department. Every day, I learned without the pressure of formal training programs and being a specialist. My enthusiasm and growing love for the specialty was rewarded with kindness and mentorship. While I never had firm plans to return, I rediscovered nuclear medicine at another career crossroads at the end of my radiology training. I reconnected with my old team, and never looked back.

One of the greatest hurdles was coming to terms with the perceived lack of patient engagement. It took me a while to admit to myself that while I loved working in oncology and palliative care and found it immensely rewarding, the emotional toll was high. I was taking my problems home to my family, which wasn't sustainable. Radiology and nuclear medicine have given me the gift of working as an oncology subspecialist in a meaningful way that suits my personality and is sustainable for me.

What do I think are the good things about a career in radiology and nuclear medicine?

I get to work in specialties that are intellectually engaging, suit my individual skills, and fulfil me. I can work flexibly in public and private settings, with my private work fully remote on a flexible schedule. I can combine it with medical education and have been able to pick up research and academic pursuits that interest me – like writing, for example. I have the privilege of working and collaborating with other like-minded people, learning from and with them every day. And at the end of the day, I enjoy it.

Advice for applications and preparing for radiology

An alternative title here would be 'preparing your resume', but I don't like to think about it this way. There is a tendency to look at preparing for radiology applications as a checkbox exercise, which degrades the spirit of why certain activities and experiences are recommended in the first place.

The experiences listed on your resume should never be considered 'one-and-done.' They should indicate the scope of skills and experience you could bring to a department and what foundational knowledge you have. It should reflect how you are preparing to be a radiology trainee, not how you are ticking the boxes so you can score an interview.

Recruiters for individual radiology programs will value certain skills and experiences differently. One site may prioritise research involvement, while another may want to know how you give back to the community outside of radiology. Some recruitment processes will be more open or blinded, and others will have more scope to prefer candidates who have established connections with the department.

It is ideal to contact the radiology department you are applying to before submitting your application. How each department manages expressions of interest is different. However, formally contacting the educational team (e.g. Directors of Training, Clinical Director or their representative) is worthwhile. Some will take the time to meet with you, others may invite you to an information night to learn more, and others still may simply record your interest. For those offered a meeting or a phone call, approach it with gratitude and listen intently. The radiologists will have given up part of their clinical day to help you and it is important that you follow through. Visiting the department in person can help give you a sense of the place and whether you would be a good fit.

It is also worthwhile speaking with current or former site trainees, both to build connections and to learn more about the realities of daily work. They may also be able to give you valuable insights into the recruitment process, which can be prepared for and incorporated into applications.

When I advise prospective trainees, I first look for evidence of **interest in and engagement with medical imaging** as a discipline. This should include experience working within a radiology or nuclear medicine department, research collaborations or mentorships with imaging specialists, and attendance at courses or conferences with a medical imaging focus (in-person or online). Given the competitive nature of training, this part of your resume must be substantial.

I suggest that their resume should also demonstrate evidence of activity and engagement in several areas:

- Research
- Teaching or academic assistance
- Quality improvement, leadership, advocacy or other healthcare initiatives
- Preparation for the anatomy and physics exams (for Australia and New Zealand)

Research is integral to evidence-based radiology and a formal part of training programs. For these reasons, research engagement and expertise are desirable. Any research outputs should be noted; however, getting involved with some medical imaging-focused projects is worthwhile. Published peer-reviewed articles should be prioritised on the written resume above conference presentations and posters.

Radiology-focused research opportunities can be scarce and competitive. To seek these out, it is best to speak with your local department or university or ask clinical supervisors to connect you with their medical imaging colleagues. You can also seek collaboration opportunities with medical imaging specialists on other projects. Suppose you wish to publish a surgical case report. If there are medical images within the case, inviting the reporting radiologist or another expert reader to help describe and annotate the findings as a co-author can help to foster connection.

Engagement with **teaching and academic assistance** can be facilitated through your clinical workplace or affiliated university. Any engagement with teaching is desirable, including bedside teaching or facilitating didactic or small-group teaching for medical students or more junior doctors. Near-peer teaching initiatives are excellent for getting started in medical education.

Being part of radiology-specific education is ideal but should be approached thoughtfully. Radiology teaching is nuanced and draws from learned experience, dedicated practice, and study. Specific imaging skills should be taught under the supervision or mentorship of more senior radiology advanced trainees or specialists.

With the shifting focus and prioritisation of professional skills through imaging training, demonstrated involvement with **quality improvement** initiatives, healthcare **leadership**, and advocacy is desirable for new trainees. This may include being part of a clinical audit, mortality and morbidity meetings, multidisciplinary team organisation, or community-based health advocacy. Potential employers are looking to see whether a candidate understands their duty as a clinician and how there is more to radiology than reading images.

For Australian and New Zealand trainees, there is an expectation that **anatomy** and **physics** (applied imaging technology) examinations will be attempted – and ideally passed – soon after commencing training. Participation in review courses should not be viewed as a checkbox that can be forgotten. Anatomy and physics are essential knowledge for commencing and continuing radiology practice.

If a practice examination has been completed, marks should be included to demonstrate your proficiency and your ability to pass the barrier exams. Passing the exams early in training will make any radiology trainees' journey easier, including providing a smoother transition into diagnostic reporting and gaining proficiency to complete after-hours shifts.

Additional professional and community involvement (including employment history, education, awards, leadership positions, etc.) should also be standard for any professional resume or application. Not all information will be appropriate, but including some extracurricular activities can add a point of interest to your application. It is best to seek local advice, as some resume inclusions may prove polarising among recruiters.

Seeking **feedback** from your local medical imaging department and other clinical mentors on your professional portfolio is helpful. They can advise you on your progress and make suggestions to fill any knowledge or experience gaps. Asking for help from radiologists can signal your interest in and dedication to them. If they make a suggestion, you should do your best to follow through. This demonstrates that you are listening and are committed. It also shows that you are serious about radiology and not there to waste their time.

Preparing for the radiology interview

Being asked to interview for a radiology training job is an indication that you are already in a good position. The recruiters are satisfied that, on paper, you could fill the role that they have vacant. As with applications, however, the interview is usually competitive.

What are interview panels looking for?

Interview formats will vary widely, and each panel will approach the process differently. At the heart of any recruitment is the desire to choose the candidate who appears to have the greatest potential to succeed as a radiology trainee in their department – in terms both of completing the requirements or training and of being a good personality fit.

An interview panel may ask themselves the following questions about potential new hires:

- Do they know enough about radiology training and practice to understand the commitment required?
- Are they capable of passing examinations and completing the mandatory training requirements?
- Will they work safely under supervision?
- Will they ask for help if required?
- Are they teachable, and will they respond maturely to feedback?
- Will they maintain consistent professional conduct while interacting with staff and patients?
- Have they taken the time to learn about radiology as a discipline and the issues facing our community?
- How will they interact with our medical imaging team?
- How will they add value to our department?
- Do I have concerns about how they would function within my department?

Consider this: recruiting a new radiology trainee in New South Wales represents a five-year commitment on behalf of the radiology department or training program. The radiologists on the panel need to be certain that the trainee they recruit will be a worthwhile investment of their time, money and emotional energy.

Preparing and presenting responses

Radiology interviews require some preparation, but should not be over-rehearsed or rigidly formulaic. Some questions will be standard, whereas others are to get to know you as a person and a doctor. Answers should come from a place of authenticity, grounded in your motivations and experiences. Interviews are not exams, but they should not be approached too casually.

In structuring responses, I suggest starting with a broad topic statement and then working from there. If you have a good idea of where your answer is going, you can add some 'signposts' e.g. 'there are *three* main reasons why I believe I would be well suited to this department. *Firstly...*' A brief summary conclusion can also help to anchor your response (depending on the nature of the question).

Most interviews will have a time limit and take you through a handful of questions. When you know the time and the number of questions, you can budget your time. For example, for a 15-minute interview with 5 questions, you would aim for approximately 2.5 minutes per question to allow buffer time for the interview to start and finish and transitions between questions.

There are some more **common interview questions** that all candidates should be able to answer well. Examples include:

- Why do you want to be a radiologist?
- Why do you want to undertake radiology training at our site?
- What makes you the right candidate for this position?
- What can you bring to this department?
- What is your understanding of the radiology training program and its requirements?
- What do you believe are the qualities of a good radiologist?

My favourite variant of these questions is: 'What have you done to prepare for radiology training?' I like this because you have the chance to judge where the candidate sees value in the experiences and achievements listed on their resume. Is preparation just about passing exams or building a resume? Or is it more about preparing yourself to be a safe and knowledgeable trainee who is well-equipped to learn and grow? I prefer those who focus on the latter, which incorporates the practical requirements of exam preparation, courses, conferences and self-directed learning.

Broad topics for other questions include:

- Basic procedural and diagnostic radiology
- Consent processes
- Adverse event management
- Communication and conflict resolution
- Quality assurance initiatives
- Research and evidence-based radiology
- Current affairs in radiology, e.g. artificial intelligence, diversity and inclusion, population-based screening
- Professional/non-interpretive skills

Particularly for **scenario-based questions**, remember who you are in the scenario. You are the radiology trainee working under supervision. There is always a more senior doctor with you who will be a point of escalation in most circumstances where things do not go according to plan. This applies to post-procedural complications, witnessing bullying from a coworker, or requiring assistance in interpreting a diagnostic study.

If you are out of your depth, go back to first principles including:

- Person-centred care & autonomy
- Basic patient assessment
- Emergency management
- Hygiene and sterile technique
- Informed consent
- Asking for help
- Treating the patient and your colleagues with respect

Questions and conclusions

A controversial note to finish. Interviewers will always ask the candidate if they have **questions**; you don't have to ask a question if you don't have any. I suggest refraining from asking the panel about things that should be assumed knowledge (e.g. how long radiology training is) or deep philosophical questions.

Whether you ask a question or not, take a moment to thank the panel for their time and give a polite sign-off. You want the panel to remember you for the right reasons.

Good luck!

ADVICE FOR APPROACHING RADIOLOGY FELLOWSHIP EXAMS

General tips for approaching radiology exams

My first foray into writing about exams and non-interpretative skills in radiology was at the invitation of *InsideRadiology*, who asked me to write some advice for those approaching exams. The exam format has changed in the six years since that was published, although much of the advice still holds true. These are my updated top seven tips for tackling exams.

1. **Report as much and as widely as possible, incorporating feedback**.
   On the whole, radiology trainees who report more in day-to-day reporting and are actively engaged with the workings of a department do better come exam day and emerge more well-rounded radiologists. Trainees who report widely have greater exposure to the broad spectrum of what is normal. They are less likely to be caught up in incidental findings and normal variation. They are more likely to detect clinically significant abnormalities, moving through cases quicker with more accuracy.

   Engaging widely with modalities will build vocabulary and familiarity with the reporting lexicon of the specific study or pathology. Using appropriate terminology improves the quality of reports. In assessments, it will signal your expertise to the examiner.

However, this advice comes with a caveat: producing large volumes of reports is not enough if you are not taking the time to receive and implement feedback. This is why adequate supervision of registrars by specialists and the provision of meaningful critique are so important. Training alone embeds your errors.

2. Build a strong support network

Radiology training is a long journey. It is often physically and intellectually draining and, at times, emotionally fraught. Medical imaging is humbling, as you are *required* to learn by making mistakes and incorporating feedback.

Your support network should include colleagues (consultants and registrars in your department), study partners and groups, and (perhaps most importantly) your friends and family. It can be too easy to lose touch with your life outside radiology while you are in the thick of exam preparation, but it is your touchstone.

Don't be afraid to ask for help when you need it. The people who care about you will gladly provide it if you let them.

3. Learn from those who have come before you

Start by asking yourself: who do you know that has been successful in the past and what can you learn from them? This includes heroes and role models, but also radiologists in your own department and those who teach you. Take note of whether there was something unique about their preparation, and listen out for pearls of hard-learned wisdom and insight. Ask them how they did it and reflect on how their advice could help you.

Success does not only mean the highest level of achievement; there is also great potential to learn from someone who has overcome difficult circumstances. One of my most admired consultants had a few attempts at a particular exam station, and now he is one of the best teachers of that system I have had the pleasure of working with. Through self-reflection and dedicated study, he became an expert. That hard-earned experience and knowledge is now there to help the next generation of radiologists.

4. Learn from those around you

When preparing exam preparation sessions, seeing the cases and working through the practice questions is only a small part of the learning experience. By reflecting on the presentation of others (as well as yourself), you can refine your presentation style and highlight gaps in your knowledge. It also helps you as an observer to stay more engaged in the session even when you aren't in the hot seat. Some questions to ask yourself include:

- What did the candidate do well?
- What did the candidate not do so well?
- Do I have knowledge gaps in this subject matter?
- Why did the examiner show this particular case? (i.e. What is the learning point?)

- How would I present this case?
- Were any pearls of wisdom in the discussion?

If you are preparing for a short-answer examination, such as the Australian and New Zealand OSCER exam, you can also brainstorm questions related to that particular imaging case to guide future study.

If you are lucky enough to attend a tutorial by an examiner or subject matter expert, keep an eye and ear out for common stumbling blocks you can address in your learning. These experts know what trips up others, and you can use this information to help prevent yourself from falling into the same trap.

5. Simulate the exam as best you can

Where possible, become familiar with the final assessment style and regularly practise in this format. The Australian and New Zealand examinations have moved away from freestyle case read-out formats to structured short-answer questions surrounding a case. This has required some tweaks to presentation style, with many preferring the new structured approach as it is less influenced by variations in a candidate's presentation style. While the descriptions of imaging observations will be similar, the trainee needs to hold back synthesis and management steps until asked, for example.

Simulation of the exam is not only about format, although this is very important. It also considers mimicking the stress and pressure of the examination. By creating unfamiliar or pressurised scenarios, you can become more comfortable in the environment that awaits you on the day of the exam. Strategies to achieve this may include:

- Presenting under time pressure
- Presenting to a larger audience
- Attending sessions with unfamiliar teachers/examiners in unfamiliar settings
- Attending formal practice examinations (with exam conditions)

Finally, the learning objectives have been authored for a reason. These will guide the creation of questions and prioritisation of important concepts. It is advisable to familiarise yourself with the scope of what could be examined so that there are no surprises waiting for you on the day.

6. Use all of the information you have been given

The medical images are only one part of the information at your disposal in an examination case – as with any clinical case reported or reviewed.

The clinical history provided can inform all stages of your approach to a case, including:

- Initial search pattern and review areas
- Assessment for causes, complications and associated findings
- Formation of a differential diagnosis list
- Recommendation of management options and follow-up

BOX 6.1   FOR EXAMPLE ...

You are in the chest/vascular station of the exam. The examiner shows a chest X-ray and gives the clinical history of:

'25-year-old woman with dull chest pain. On clinical examination there is distension of the neck veins.'

Before reviewing the case, some potential differential diagnoses are considered based on the clinical history e.g. a mediastinal mass or large thoracic mass compressing the thoracic inlet. When the case is reviewed, the search can start with the mediastinal outline and lung apices.

The case shows a mediastinal contour abnormality concerning for a mass.

Anterior mediastinal masses are more common in younger patients, with lymphoma the most common cause in young females ahead of thymic neoplasms and germ cell neoplasms. This knowledge will help assess for findings specific to these lesions and order the differential diagnosis list.

If you have forgotten the clinical history under pressure from the exam, you can ask for it again. It is better to ask than to continue in the wrong direction.

7. Take care of yourself

This is one of the most important pieces of advice I can give you, and the hardest to follow. At times during my training and examination preparation I did a horrible job of this. Be kind to yourself and allow time for sleep, rest and downtime. Ask for help and connect with your general practitioner or other mental health support services if needed. Remember that radiology training and assessments are not easy, and *everyone* struggles (regardless of whether they appear to or not). No-one completes exams perfectly and everyone makes mistakes.

Burnout is highly prevalent in doctors – especially trainees – and it is important to know the signs to recognise them in yourself. I recommend visiting theburnoutproject.com.au to learn more.

Preparing for and presenting questions on intrinsic roles

Questions on *Intrinsic Roles* (professionalism and non-interpretive skills) account for 5% of the RANZCR final oral exam – the OSCER. (Objective Structured Clinical Examination in Radiology) Across each of the subspecialty stations, this equates to 1–2 such questions coming up in each exam station. Each question will be supported by a marking rubric or answer key, meaning that there will be essential information that needs to be conveyed to the examiner to be awarded a passing grade.

The OSCER has been designed as a capstone exam, meaning that it should (in theory) be testing knowledge that reflects the training journey of the junior doctor as they work towards becoming a specialised radiologist. These questions should test knowledge and experiential skills beyond what a sensible medical student, intern or resident should know.

Intrinsic Role competencies are the professional skills the community would consider a 'good' radiologist to have. Clinical radiologists require these skills to deliver safe and effective healthcare to our community and work effectively within the collaborative team-based environment of modern healthcare. The importance of culturally safe and inclusive practice cannot be understated, particularly regarding overcoming healthcare inequities and the importance of considering the needs of First People in practice. Expect these topics to be examined.

As with any exam, preparation, planning, knowledge gathering, and practice will be key. You might find printing and annotating the outcomes a good way to think through and brainstorm questions, either by yourself or with your study group. When you are in case-based tutorials, take a moment to think if an Intrinsic Role question could fit into the scenario.

BOX 6.2   FOR EXAMPLE ...

You have just described the findings and recommended management options for a CT case demonstrating a new diagnosis of metastatic colorectal cancer.

Here are some example intrinsic role questions which could relate to this case scenario:

- *Outline the role the Colorectal Cancer Multidisciplinary Team could have in managing this patient.*
- *The patient has arrived prior for an ultrasound guided liver biopsy. She does not speak English and appears frightened. How would you approach the consent process in this patient?*
- *Suppose the patient is of Aboriginal or Māori heritage. Outline the role cultural support staff (e.g. Liaison Officers) could have during the patient's engagement with the radiology department.*
- *You wonder whether the administration of oral contrast would improve diagnostic accuracy for patients with suspected bowel cancer. Briefly, how would you design an audit to assess this?*

When deriving intrinsic role questions, you can see that there are some overarching concepts and themes that can be applied to various scenarios. The value of a multidisciplinary team can be considered across different oncology subspecialties, chronic diseases and complex presentations. Cultural safety is important for all patients (especially those from Indigenous communities), and can therefore be asked in any OSCER station. Quality assurance/improvement and research are the backbone of evidence-based radiology, and questions about these topics are also widely applicable. Some concepts may be subspecialty or condition-specific, such as managing non-accidental injury detection in paediatrics or ethical issues specific to women's imaging.

When structuring answers, particularly those that require more in-depth discussion, I like to draw inspiration from my high school debating training.

Start with a broad introductory statement, which orientates yourself and signals to the examiner that you are across the subject matter. If you have the information at hand, you can provide a brief summary of the salient points. This serves two purposes: firstly, it helps you to organise your thoughts and express your competency, and secondly if you run out of time you may be able to score yourself some marks at the outset.

After this, briefly, clearly and logically describe the components of your answer, being sure to note any high-yield facts and terms.

A brief concluding statement can be helpful to round out your discussion and signal your completion.

BOX 6.3   FOR EXAMPLE …

Question: How are patient safety incidents classified? Provide some examples from radiology.

Incidents in healthcare are considered when an unplanned or unintended event arises which has the potential to or does result in patient care.

There are three types of patient safety incidents: harmful incidents (or adverse events), 'no harm' incidents, and near-misses.

Harmful incidents are when the event results in direct harm to the patient. An example in radiology is performing a lung biopsy of the wrong pulmonary nodule.

A 'no harm' event is when an event occurred but no harm was caused to the patient. An example may be if a 10mm adrenal adenoma was not reported on an imaging study. The lesion appeared stable when it was detected and reported on a subsequent examination 1 year later.

A near-miss can also be termed a 'close call'. It occurs when a potential hazard or error is identified and corrected before the event can occur. An example of this would be a request form asking for an X-ray of the right arm to follow up on a fracture when the injury was on the left. The radiographer checked the injury site with the patient, and the correct side was imaged.

Acknowledging and managing patient safety incidents in radiology practice is essential to delivering high-quality person-centred care, regardless of whether harm is directly caused.

My general tips for tackling the OSCER exam

Listen to the question

Listen to what your examiner is asking and respond to the specific question. If you have been asked for 'observations', time could be wasted by exploring a long differential diagnosis list or debating the appropriate management plan. Describe the salient abnormalities and pull the findings together. Then, wait for the next question.

Focus in on the abnormality

Depending on how the case images are presented, that is, as a series or static image, your approach and search strategy will need to be adapted. For a scrollable stack, you will naturally need to give yourself a couple of seconds to find the abnormality and home in on it – but don't spend too much time doing this. For a single captured image, the abnormality usually becomes apparent quickly.

Your practice and preparation must encompass drilled search strategies and pattern recognition. These will vary based on pathologies and modalities, but they should be designed to extract the information that is clinically important for the patient.

Get to the point

In the old exam format, I strongly advocated talking to give yourself 'thinking time' at the beginning. This would involve repeating the history and clarifying the exam before you, giving you time to examine the case and get your bearings. There is less time for 'throat-clearing' exercises in the short answer formats.

You can give yourself a few seconds to orientate yourself, which should be no more than one or two deep breaths. After this, candidates need to get the pertinent findings out quickly. For each case, focus on the high-yield and relevant facts, as these are the ones that will win you the most marks and drive the case forward.

It is useful to ask how you would handle this particular case if you encountered it in the real world under time pressure:

> *If I were on a busy shift and I had 30 seconds to tell the emergency doctor what was happening on the scan, what would I say?*

Do not feel that you need to 'earn' the right to look at all the information you have been given e.g. you should look at both the frontal and lateral chest X-rays as you describe, rather than describing the frontal film entirely before moving on.

You should quickly review the provided images as you start your presentation. A classic example is a hypersensitivity pneumonitis case. The expiratory phase CT will almost always hold the definitive answer, allowing the radiology trainee to move through the case quickly if they recognise the pattern of air trapping. However, a candidate may be tempted to spend too much time on the inspiratory CT phase before moving on. This can eat into valuable time.

Streamlining your presentation

In a generic sense, I suggest starting with the *'what'* and *'where'* to craft a broad topic sentence. This orientates you and will help later in forming differential diagnoses.

BOX 6.4   FOR EXAMPLE …

Examples of opening statements to orientate you and the examiners:

- *There is a large parenchymal lesion in the left frontal lobe, causing mass effect.*
- *There is a pleural abnormality in the left hemithorax.*
- *There is an aggressive lesion centred at the distal metaphysis of the right femur.*
- *There is large volume pneumoperitoneum.*

After starting your presentation with the salient abnormality, you can move through the characterisation of the finding and problem-solving. This may encompass a '**causes, complications, associated findings**' approach; pair this with a **staging classification** in the setting of malignancy (tumour, nodes, metastases), or conduct a **systematic appraisal** e.g. when assessing a trauma scan.

Having a structure to describe the case can also serve the candidate well under pressure and improve daily reporting accuracy and speed.

Causes, complications, associated findings

'Causes, complications and associated findings' is a personal mantra of mine. Even medical students can point out an abnormality and say, 'There's the problem'. Where we add value as radiologists is considering the abnormality in its context:

- Cause:
  - Can I see the cause somewhere on this scan?
  - Is there something in the clinical history that will give me a clue to the cause?
  - Can this information help me narrow down my differential diagnosis?
- Complications:
  - How does the abnormality affect the surrounding environment in the body?
  - What review areas should I check for complications associated with this abnormality?
  - Can I screen complications on the series I have been given, or do I need more information?
- Associated findings:
  - Is this condition associated with other manifestations, and could they be present on these images?
  - Does the patient require other imaging or clinical tests?

If you see a lung mass, for example, you could apply this framework as follows:

- Are there features of smoking-related lung disease? (Cause)
- Is there bronchial obstruction/post-obstructive bronchiectasis? Is there vascular invasion or pulmonary emboli? (Complications)
- Is there evidence of nodal or visceral metastases? (Associated findings)

The more practised this approach (or your chosen approach) is, the more streamlined your presentation will become. It is also a good way to consider whether you need to include relevant negatives, which can be challenging inboth the exam setting and daily reporting.

BOX 6.5 FOR EXAMPLE ...

A lung mass is detected on a CT of the thorax.

Causes:

*   Are there features of smoking-related lung disease?
*   Is there evidence of asbestos exposure or occupational lung disease?

Complications:

*   Is the tumour invading local structures?
*   Is there bronchial obstruction/post-obstructive bronchiectasis?
*   Is there vascular invasion or pulmonary emboli?

Associated findings:

*   Is there evidence of nodal or visceral metastases?

Close it out

A brief conclusion is helpful if your presentation extends beyond 20 seconds or a few short sentences. This should be succinct and avoid repetition of long descriptions. If you have been solely asked for your observations, you could conclude a more complex anterior mediastinal case like this: "In summary, there is a large heterogeneously enhancing anterior mediastinal mass with associated mediastinal lymphadenopathy."

If the diagnosis is unequivocal, you could offer it at this stage (depending on the case). If there is a long differential list, holding back pending the examiner's next question may be best.

When you have concluded your presentation, you can signal to your examiner with a pause. The next question or case will arise, and you can continue demonstrating your hard-earned knowledge and skills to the examiners.

Final thoughts

Remember that you are more than the exam.
You often cannot see how far you have come or how good you are.
Everyone misses cases in tutorials, but it does not make you a poor exam candidate.
Everyone misses cases in exams, but it does not mean you will fail the exam.
Even if you don't pass the exam, it does not mean you won't be a good radiologist.
Exam results do not reflect who you are as a person.
Good luck, and take care of yourself.

Index

Pages in *italics* refer to figures, pages in **bold** refer to tables, and pages followed by "n" refer to notes.

A

abuse and neglect, witnessing and identifying, 80–81
accountability
 mutual, 39
 personal, 40–41
accuracy, calculation of, 117
ACR Appropriateness Criteria®, 75–76
active learning, 89–90
active listening, 4
adverse events
 documenting, 17
 managing, 13–14
aggression, managing, 29–30, **30**
allyship, 35–36
analytical studies, 105
anchoring bias, 18
artificial intelligence (AI), 137
 applications in radiology, **138**, 140
 circumstantial challenges, 139–140
 intrinsic challenges, 139
assessment, 8–9
 targeted, 9–10
attributable risk, 109
attribution bias, 18

B

barriers to healthcare
 for people living with disabilities, 133
 for rural and remote populations, 132–133
bias, 126
 in radiology research, 102–103; *see also*
  cognitive biases
Bloom's *Taxonomy of Educational Objectives*, **87**
bullying, 44
burnout, 92–93, 153
 in radiologists, **93**
 strategies for reducing, *94*

C

CanMEDs Framework, xi
case-control studies, 106
categorical data, 114

Chi-square test, 115
Choosing Wisely, 76–77
clinical audit, 72–73
clinical meetings, *see* multidisciplinary meetings
  (MDMs)
clinical question, formulating, 120
clinical reference standard, 122
clinician well-being and wellness, 91–92
Closing the Gap report, 128
Cochrane Collaboration, 107
cognitive biases, 18
cohort studies, 105
communication
 with anxious patients, 28–29
 in conflict, 48
 and cultural safety, 130–131
 of diagnostic certainty, 21–22
 errors, 26
 of findings, life-threatening or clinically
  significant, 23
 and language difficulties, 27
 mismatch with health literacy, 27
 and person-centred care, 3
 types in radiology, 1–2
communication breakdown, between medical staff,
  46–47
comparison imaging, locating and reviewing, 16
complications
 documenting, 17
 managing, 13–14
confidence interval, 115
confidentiality, 79–80
 in medical research, 101
confirmation bias, 18
conflict, 43
 personal communication in, 48
 principles for managing, 47–48
conflicts of interest, 81
conscious bias, 126
consultation, 8–9
 targeted, 9–10
continuing medical education (CME), 83
continuing professional development (CPD), 83
continuous variables, 114
counselling, 10–11

Printed in the United States
by Baker & Taylor Publisher Services